# Descending with angels

MANCHESTER
1824

Manchester University Press

**Anthropology, Creative Practice and Ethnography (ACE)**

*Series editors*: Faye Ginsburg, Paul Henley, Andrew Irving and Sarah Pink

*Previously published*

David MacDougall, *The looking machine: Essays on cinema, anthropology and documentary filmmaking*

*Forthcoming titles*

Paul Henley, *Beyond observation: A history of authorship in ethnographic film*

In association with the Granada Centre for Visual Anthropology

# Descending with angels

## Islamic exorcism and psychiatry: a film monograph

CHRISTIAN SUHR

Manchester University Press

Published by Manchester University Press
Altrincham Street, Manchester M1 7JA

www.manchesteruniversitypress.co.uk

British Library Cataloguing-in-Publication Data
A catalogue record for this book is available from the British Library

ISBN 978 1 5261 4031 9 hardback
ISBN 978 1 5261 4591 8 paperback

First published 2019



Typeset in Bembo
by Toppan Best-set Premedia Limited
Printed in Great Britain
by TJ International Ltd, Padstow

*With every raindrop there is an angel who descends with it until he places it where God has ordered.*

Hadith reported by al-Tabari,
narrated by al-Hakam ibn Utayba and Hasan al-Basri

# Contents

# List of film scenes

*Descending with angels*, ethnographic documentary, 75 min.
Filmed and edited by Christian Suhr, Persona Film, 2013.

For readers of this book, the film *Descending with angels* can be accessed at the website www.descendingwithangels.com with the password: ruqya.

To purchase the film for public or classroom use contact
Documentary Educational Resources
Phone: (617) 926-0491 | orders@der.org | www.der.org.

1 Rain at night-time, Aarhus Vest, prayer in the mosque (*qiyām al-layl*).
2 Shaykh Abu Bilal exorcising a jinn, Abu Omar's apartment: 2:59.
3 Noon prayer (*ṣalāt al-ẓuhr*) performed by Nour Aziz who then explains his problems with magic and psychiatry: 11:38.
4 Monthly meeting: Aziz discusses his illness with his psychiatrist Jørgen Aagaard, Aarhus University Hospital, Risskov: 15:32.
5 Abu Bilal examines a young woman for possession by jinn: 21:16.
6 Esther Isaksen, Jørgen Aagaard, and Christian Suhr watch and discuss the film recordings, Aarhus University Hospital, Risskov: 29:21.
7 Young Muslims watch and discuss a YouTube video entitled '7000 year old jinn inside man', Brabrand: 32:59.
8 Weekly meeting: Aziz discusses his condition and the effects of psychotropic medication with his nurse Esther, Aarhus University Hospital, Risskov: 40:52.
9 Abu Bilal and Christian watch the film recordings: Abu Bilal explains his views on illness and psychotropic medication: 44:59.
10 Lecture about Quranic healing in the mosque, Society for Equality and Brotherhood, Brabrand: 48:04.
11 Esther and Christian discuss the exorcism of Abu Omar and reasons why the jinn did not speak: 51:25.
12 Abu Bilal, Abu Bashir, Umm Omar, and Abu Omar evaluate the exorcism of Abu Omar's jinn and Abu Bilal performs additional reading: 53:57.
13 Esther and Christian talk about the possible dangers of exorcism and psychiatry. Esther argues for the necessity of care in healing: 1:03:27.
14 Monthly meeting: Jørgen, Esther, and Birte Gam explain the necessity of continued medication to Aziz and also acknowledge the healing effect of Aziz's religious practice: 1:05:32.
15 Evening prayer during Ramadan (*ṣalāt al-tarāwīḥ*): 1:13:38.

# List of figures

# Series editors' preface

Anthropology, Creative Practice and Ethnography provides a forum for authors and practitioners from across the digital humanities and social sciences to explore the rapidly developing opportunities offered by visual, acoustic and textual media for generating ethnographic understandings of social, cultural and political life. It addresses both established and experimental fields of visual anthropology, including film, photography, sensory and acoustic ethnography, ethnomusicology, graphic anthropology, digital media and other creative modes of representation. The series features works that engage in the theoretical and practical interrogation of the possibilities and constraints of audiovisual media in ethnographic research, while simultaneously offering a critical analysis of the cultural, political and historical contexts.

We were delighted to launch the series with David MacDougall's *The looking machine*: a new and important collection of essays by one of the world's leading ethnographic filmmakers and writers on cinema. We are equally pleased to follow this with Christian Suhr's *Descending with angels*. This book offers an in-depth discussion of the many different issues raised by a feature-length, award-winning, ethnographic film of the same name, now available on-line, that Suhr made as part of his research on Islamic exorcism and psychiatry. In articulating film with text, *Descending with angels* addresses in a direct fashion our interest in using this series to explore the ways in which different media may be combined to produce fuller and more rounded ethnographic accounts.

Other works by senior figures in visual anthropology and film are currently in production. We are also keen to encourage submissions from new authors from a broad diversity of backgrounds, including those from outside the English-speaking world. We very much look forward to hearing from authors interested in contributing to this collective adventure in contemporary ethnographic representation.

Paul Henley and Andrew Irving
Granada Centre for Visual Anthropology, University of Manchester

# A guide to the book and film

THIS book includes a feature-length ethnographic film produced as part of my research on Islamic exorcisms and psychiatry in Denmark. The film introduces the reader to the dynamics of possession and psychosis through concrete examples of the interactions between Quranic healers, Muslim patients, and psychiatrists. The film scenes act as catalysts for questions I then analyse and discuss in the chapters of the book. In addition the film provides a form of analysis in its own right, allowing insights into emotional and existential dilemmas among both patients and healers that complement the written analysis but also invite the reader to think beyond the conclusions of the book. Jinn possession and psychosis are concepts that describe essentially invisible forms of suffering. Taken together, the book and film explore the possibilities of juxtaposing text with film material which, in combination, may create a space for the invisible in scholarly analysis. I recommend watching the film before reading the book (see p. viii for online access). In addition I invite the reader to revisit individual scenes as they are referenced throughout the chapters. Below I provide an overview of the topics and the arguments addressed in the chapters of the book and how they might be read together with the film.

I begin the book by outlining how the invisible has been dealt with in the social sciences, in Islamic theology, and in public debates in Western media on the question of whether Islam is in fact the underlying invisible cause of 'integration problems'. My exploration of the invisibility and hypervisibility of Muslims in the West leads to a discussion of invisibility in relation to theories about human perceptual agency. While a number of influential studies in anthropology and psychiatry have been concerned with how best to account for human agency, I suggest that both psychiatric treatments and Islamic healing point primarily to the idea of human agency as an obstacle that needs to be overcome in order to access either the invisible healing of God, or that of psychotropic medicine. Finally I discuss my approach to ethnographic film and how I have applied the cinematic gaze as a methodological and analytical tool for displacing my own perception when studying the invisible among Danish Muslims.

The second chapter begins with a discussion of recent anthropological debates about how to take the viewpoints of others seriously, even when doing so implies accepting the existence of invisible beings and phenomena such as angels, jinn, God, schizophrenia, psychosis, or depression. I describe a number of critical experiences and conversations with interlocutors that occurred during the course of my engagement with this project. In the chapter, I also introduce several of the people in the film, including Nour Aziz and his nurse Esther Isaksen at the psychiatric hospital in Risskov (Scenes 3, 8, and 14) and Shaykh Abu Bilal (Scenes 2, 5, 9, 10, and 12) as he tries to exorcise a jinn spirit. In addition, I discuss the methodological and personal dilemmas of conducting long-term anthropological fieldwork in a highly politicised context.

In the third chapter, I analyse Scene 7, which provides an example of how young Muslims use the increasing number of jinn exorcisms on YouTube as a form of entertainment, but also as a way of cultivating an awareness and an ethical disposition of the self in confrontation with the invisible. I describe how these exorcisms produce doubt and discuss the ways in which doubt is an integral part of these young Muslims' practices of faith. In addition I explore how the recurrent discussion of the value of images in anthropology could find new answers by examining the way these Muslims use and respond to visual media. In conclusion I point out how the visual display of the photographic image shares a peculiar resemblance with the bodies of people possessed by invisible jinn. Like the possessed body, the image as a failed example or model of reality makes certain things visible, but simultaneously amplifies the sense of invisibility, pointing towards that which cannot be seen, depicted visually, or represented in writing. This suggests a negative epistemology in which images obtain their value not from the adequacy of their correspondence to perceived reality, but rather from the ways in which they fail to exemplify that which they appear to depict.

Chapter 4 takes a further step into the specific healing interactions between Muslim patients, psychiatrists, and Quranic healers by introducing the story of Feisal, whom I met during my fieldwork when he was going through a long series of exorcisms. In addition I take a close look at Scene 5 in which a young woman is being diagnosed for jinn possession and Scene 6 in which I discuss the film recordings of the young woman together with the nurse Esther Isaksen and the psychiatrist Jørgen Aagaard. I analyse how Islamic exorcisms and psychiatric healthcare depend on an oscillation between making visible and keeping invisible – between giving a tangible visual form to the suffering of patients and to possible paths for their healing, and yet simultaneously disabling and dismantling other possible visualisations. Iconoclastic practices in both psychiatric healthcare and Islamic exorcism are related to the issue of faith in healing and the necessity of doubt in order to attain faith. Both in psychiatric encounters and in Islamic exorcisms, an effort is made to produce doubt as the condition for submission in faith to the healing agent. Here the widely disputed notion of 'patient' is of key importance. In contrast to recent user-oriented and holistic approaches in psychiatry, as well as a number of studies in medical anthropology that tend to emphasise healing as an effect of human self-creativity, the issue in the treatments I studied was not framed in terms of how to gain agency; rather, the main concern was 'how to become a patient', which involved the surrender of individual agency in favour of allowing something else to do the work of healing.

The fifth chapter explores the sacrifices expected from patients in both systems of treatment. Taking the near-sacrifice of Abraham's son as a model for healing, I explore the ways in which patients – through leaps of faith – dismantle those parts within themselves perceived by the healer as the core of their suffering: psychotic delusions, jinn, or the desires of what in Islamic theology is referred to as the lower self. In conclusion I argue that self-sacrifice of this kind enables the patients to submit to their treatment, and thereby to be reinstated as moral and healthy subjects in the structural order implied by the two systems of healing: biomedicine and Salafi-oriented interpretations of Islam. The chapter expands on the analysis of Scenes 5 and 6 presented in Chapter 4, but also explores the interaction between Aziz and his psychiatrist as seen in Scenes 3 and 4.

Chapter 6 moves on to describe the aesthetic forms applied in the healing encounters in order to facilitate the possibility of self-sacrifice, and to move beyond the boundaries of the immediately visible. I explore the healing encounters as ritual events that aim at the dissolution of the subject. Inspired by recent attempts to apply the film theory of Eisenstein, Vertov, and Deleuze to the theorisation of ritual and religious art, I analyse the exorcism of Abu Omar (in Scenes 2 and 12) and the treatment of Aziz by his nurse Esther (in Scenes 8 and 14) as a ritual dialectic moving towards dissolution by way of disruptive montage. I conclude that submission to a particular form of healing is facilitated by the healers' ability to conjure the sense of an all-encompassing world of knowledge and total vision to which the patients' limited and partial perspectives must subject themselves.

The final chapter of the book concludes on the findings of the preceding chapters, and critically discusses to what extent the analysis as a whole has adequately accounted for the work of the invisible in Islamic and psychiatric healing. If the invisible is indeed invisible, as claimed both by existential phenomenologists like Maurice Merleau-Ponty and Emmanuel Levinas, as well as in Islamic theology, it would be problematic if my weaving in and out of Islamic exorcisms and Danish psychiatry had succeeded in outlining and visualising the work of the invisible in any finite or exhaustive way. For this reason I have dedicated the final chapter of the book to those aspects of the treatments that – as pockets of still unexplored invisibility – stubbornly refuse to fit within the analytical scheme of the book.

# Note on translation, transliteration, and informed consent

THE fieldwork for this research and film project was carried out in a mixture of Danish, Arabic, and English. While most sermons and prayers in the mosques of Aarhus would be conducted in classical Arabic with occasional translations into Danish, many of the conversations between my interlocutors often occurred in a combination of Danish, English, and colloquial Arabic (mainly Palestinian and Iraqi dialects). While some of the people I worked with speak Arabic fluently, many of my Afghan, Somali, and Turkish interlocutors, and some of the young Arabs, often preferred to speak in Danish. My language skills allowed me to understand and identify the main content of sermons and conversations in Arabic, but many of the details I have had translated subsequently with the kind help of people from the mosques.

Throughout the chapters and the film I have translated both Danish and Arabic quotations into English. When meanings of particular words could be interpreted in divergent ways I have included original phrases in parentheses. In addition many of the standard Islamic greetings, supplications, and concepts such as *siḥr* (magic) or *khushūʿ* (humility) have been kept in Arabic to convey the flavour of the communication, which often fluctuated indistinctly between the different linguistic registers.

For the transliteration of Arabic words and phrases I generally adopted the system outlined in the *International Journal of Middle East Studies*. For ease of reading I have omitted diacritical marks for place names, proper names, and the names of my interlocutors. For words such as Quran, hadith, or the category of invisible spirits called jinn I have used their customary English spelling. Rather than distinguishing between *jinn* (plural), *jinnī* (singular masculine), and *jinnīyya* (singular feminine), I use jinn in both singular and plural as is common in English (*Oxford English Dictionary* 2013). For Quranic verses I generally use M. A. S. Abdel Haleem's (2005) translation. In addition I sometimes rely on translations and interpretations of particular Quranic concepts provided by my interlocutors in the mosques. In subtitling the film, many of the Quranic verses and Islamic supplications have been severely shortened and abridged in order to ease viewing.

When people have explicitly asked to remain anonymous or when I have judged it necessary to keep the identities of particular individuals private, their names and backgrounds have been changed. In the film I have concealed the identity of a number of people through the editing and framing of images. The people who do appear with their own names in the film and book have all been informed about the scope and aims of the research project and have explicitly given their consent. After a number of preliminary screenings of the film and discussions of the written text, I have adjusted the editing and writing according to the requests of those who appear in it.

My interlocutors in the mosques and in Danish psychiatry all had their own, and sometimes conflicting, reasons for participating in this research project. Some nurses and psychiatrists expressed a strong need for more knowledge about the treatment of Muslim patients. Furthermore some expressed a wish to demystify and illustrate how psychiatric encounters actually take place. Similarly, among the people I worked with in the mosques, many expressed a wish to show a side of their religious practice that seldom reaches public debates about Islam in the West. Some participated in the project in the hope that it might highlight something of the truth or strength of Islam, and perhaps even become a form of *daʿwa* (invitation to Islam). I have attempted to take all of these desires and requests seriously so as to establish the research process as a collaborative project. Therefore it is my interlocutors' interpretations and translations of their own practices that provide the starting point for my analysis. Yet I am painfully aware that the book and film fulfil only to a very limited degree the ambitions of all my interlocutors. The book and film present my best efforts to provide a fair account of the religious and psychiatric treatments experienced by patients. Any responsibility for flaws, biases, and omissions within the analysis is entirely mine.

# Acknowledgements

THIS book and film was made possible by kind permission of the Society for Equality and Brotherhood in Brabrand, Aarhus Vest, and the Centre South and Team for Transcultural Psychiatry at Aarhus University Hospital, Risskov. I wish to thank first and foremost all the people – shaykhs, ordinary mosquegoers, nurses, social workers, psychiatrists, and other health professionals – who invited me in and attempted to help me understand their views on the healing practices they engaged in. Most of all, I owe thanks to the patients being treated in the psychiatric institutions and the mosques, and to their relatives. Their trust and willingness to share their experiences despite difficult circumstances taught me a lesson about the human capacity for hospitality, patience, and for continuing to hope even when life is at its most unbearable. Most of the patients have remained anonymous in this book and film. I wish especially to thank Nour Aziz and Abu Omar, who agreed to participate in this project with their real names and faces.

I owe special thanks to Shaykh Abu Bilal, who supported and believed in the value of this project from beginning to end. Among the people in the mosques, I also want to thank Shaykh Abu Khalid and his family, who initially invited me to conduct this film and research project in Brabrand, and Abu Bashir, who patiently sat with me for so many hours translating sermons and conversations exceeding my level of Arabic.

Feisal, Sara, Nadia, Erdam, Khalid, Abu Abdallah, Abdel Rahman, and Abu Samir are the pseudonyms of people who entrusted me with their stories. I am deeply grateful to all of you. A very special thanks to Feisal with whom I shared many ups and downs and to Abu Samir, who taught me a great deal about the anthropological method of participant observation by inviting me to take part in prayer. I also thank Adrees, Hassan, Rene, Imad, Mubarak, Karzan, Chya, Abdel Nasir, Mustafa, Mufit, Khalil, Abu Muhammad, and Abu Suleiman who spent time explaining their understanding of Islamic theology; and Said, for our discussions about film and the aesthetic qualities of the Quran. In addition I wish to warmly thank Umm Omar, Liliane Hajjou, Sami Saidana, and Naveed Baig for advice and guidance.

At Centre South at the Aarhus University Hospital in Risskov, I owe thanks first and foremost to Esther Isaksen and Jørgen Aagaard. Much of the analysis presented in this book has emerged through continued discussion with Esther and Jørgen at the hospital, and with Abu Bilal and Abu Samir in the mosque. Both Esther and Jørgen kindly agreed to appear on film, and both subsequently added a number of new perspectives on the film material that I was not able to see myself. Furthermore Jørgen acted as a voluntary supervisor in guiding me through the ethics of conducting research among mentally ill patients, and in supplying me with literature on topics such as voice-hearing, psycho-education, and the foundational psychological processes of the human mind. A large part of the fieldwork was also carried out among the nurses and psychiatrists at the Team for Transcultural Psychiatry. Here I especially wish to thank Lili Bermann and Dina Elsenoussy. Furthermore I wish to thank Birte Gam from Aarhus Municipality who has been Aziz's social worker for many years.

Writing this book would not have been possible without the assistance of Rane Willerslev, Ton Otto, and Mark Sedgwick. I wish to thank Rane for being such a constant source of inspiration and for having ambitions on behalf of this project that far exceeded what I felt capable of. Many of the conclusions presented in this book about ethnographic film and its relationship to the invisible stem from our joint readings of montage theory and phenomenology. I wish to thank Ton, who was immensely helpful in setting up this project and provided me with necessary revisions while writing the book. Ton taught me most of what I know about ethnographic fieldwork during our previous film projects in the Manus province of Papua New Guinea. Last but not least I thank Mark, whose expertise on Islam and careful instructions have guided me through the project from its initial conception to the final stages. I also wish to thank him for being there at a time when fieldwork had become too challenging for me.

For readings and corrections of the book manuscript at various stages of the process I am deeply grateful to Carolina Sanchez Boe, Amira Mittermaier, Martijn van Beek, Laura U. Marks, Michaela Schäuble, and Jennifer Deger – without your thoughtful input, criticisms, and constructive suggestions this book would not have been the same. In addition I owe special thanks to Andreas Bandak, Nadia Fadil, and Kasper Mathiesen, who have been intellectual soulmates in the process of writing, and who also have contributed with highly needed criticism to several parts of the book. For helping me through the very last revisions I warmly thank Chris Wright.

At the Department of Anthropology at Aarhus University I wish to thank my colleagues for providing such a generous environment for learning and producing anthropology and especially Mikkel Rytter, Lotte Meinert, Jens Seeberg, Mette-Louise Johansen, Nanna Schneidermann, Thomas Fibiger, Bjarke Nielsen, Thea Skaanes, Henrik Hvenegaard, Steffen Dalsgaard, Andreas Gadeberg, Marie Louise Tørring, Bodil Selmer, Nils Bubandt, Noa Vaisman, Morten Nielsen, Anne-Line Dalsgaard, Poul Pedersen, and Mohammad Bandar for valuable comments.

In the production of the film I benefited greatly from the encouragement and suggestions of Jakob and Arine Høgel, Christian Vium, Karen Waltorp, and Joe Bini. Furthermore I wish to thank Daniela Vavrova, Tove Nyholm, Paul Stoller, Nikolas Rose, Simon O'Meara, Lene Kühle, Cheryl Mattingly, Jennifer Cool, Berit Madsen, Sasha Rubel, Mayanthi Fernando, Peter Crawford, Jens Kreinath, and Martha Reineke who provided important input in the making of the film and book. At the Adorno Studios at Aarhus University I wish to thank Allan Nielsen for the many cups of coffee, joyful conversations, and for providing editing facilities in the production of the film. Anders Clausen, Kirstine Sinclair, Hjarn von Zernichow Borberg, Vibeke Borberg, and Niels Valdemar Vinding – who participated with me in some difficult public debates over the last years – I am grateful for the way you have sharpened my understanding of Danish integration politics.

As part of the research process I was offered the opportunity to spend six months at the Department of Anthropology at the University of California in Berkeley. I am deeply grateful to Charles Hirschkind for inviting me and for his help with my project. In addition I also wish to thank the late Saba Mahmood; Laura Nader; and Susan Ervin-Tripp who all provided invaluable input to the book and film. I am especially grateful to Stefania Pandolfo, who read and commented on the manuscript and whose research and teaching has been a constant source of inspiration in the development of the analysis. In the research community at Berkeley I also thank Patricia Kubala, Sultan Doughan, Himali Dixit, Antony Pattathu, and Merissa Nathan Gerson. Not least I wish to thank Bruno Reinhardt, for sharing so many of his cigarettes and so much of his vast knowledge of anthropology with me.

I owe great thanks to Lucy Seton-Watson and Melissa Brakel for revising the manuscript and the subtitles of the film and to Lucy for correcting my Arabic translation and transliteration. In Egypt, where this project started in 2005, I owe special thanks to Ashraf Abu Zuba and his family, Hanan Shawky, Shaykh Desuqi, and the late Said Subki for patiently explaining to me the role of jinn and the invisible in the lives of Muslims.

The study was jointly funded by Knud Højgaard's Foundation, the Danish Ministry for Innovation and Science, the Aarhus University research programme 'Camera as Cultural Critique', EpiCenter, Aarhus University Research Foundation, and the Danish Council for Independent Research (DFF-1321-00169). It was hosted by Moesgaard Museum and the School of Culture and Society at Aarhus University. At these institutions I thank Bjarke Paarup and Jan Skamby for their support in the overall plans to develop a centre for Visual Anthropology at Moesgaard, of which this project was a part.

I also wish to thank the editors of the Manchester University Press book series 'Anthropology, Creative Practice and Ethnography', Andrew Irving and Paul Henley; my commissioning editor, Thomas Dark;

Humairaa Dudhwala; and my copy-editor, Muhammad Ridwaan, for their help with the book, as well as the publishers of a number of journals in which parts of the chapters have been presented for allowing me to reproduce revised versions of these sections in this book.

Some of my ideas about the invisible and its relation to film have in a different form been published in the article 'Can film show the invisible: The work of montage in ethnographic filmmaking', Suhr and Willerslev, *Current Anthropology*, 53(3), 2012, pp. 282–94 (reprinted by permission of Chicago University Press). Some of my reflections on faith and the ontological turn in Chapter 2 have been published in the article 'Is there a place for faith in anthropology: Religion, reason, and the ethnographer's divine revelation', Willerslev and Suhr, *HAU: Journal of Ethnographic Theory*, 8(1–2), 2018, pp. 65–78 (reprinted by permission of Chicago University Press). My analysis of the young men watching YouTube exorcisms in Chapter 3 has in a different form appeared in 'The failed image and the possessed: Examples of invisibility in visual anthropology and Islam', *Journal of the Royal Anthropological Institute*, 21(1), 2015, pp. 96–112 (reprinted by permission of John Wiley and Sons). Parts of the analysis in Chapter 6 have appeared in the article 'Islamic exorcism and the cinema fist: Analyzing exorcism among Danish Muslims through the prism of film,' *Contemporary Islam*, 2017 (reprinted by permission of Springer Nature, https://doi.org/10.1007/s11562-017-0394-6). The discussion about Umm Omar's tripod in Chapter 6 also appears in the article 'Camera monologue: Cultural critique beyond collaboration, participation and dialogue', *Journal of Visual Anthropology*, 31, 2018, pp. 376–93 (reprinted by permission of Taylor & Francis Ltd, www.tandfonline.com).

In addition to all these people and institutions I wish to thank both of my parents, Lone Suhr and Carsten Nielsen, and their two sets of families, as well as my mother-in-law, Grethe Bahnsen, for all their help and understanding. To my wife, Mette Bahnsen, and to my sons Asger and Laurits: I do not know how to express how grateful I am for your support, guidance, and criticisms, and for the way you have provided me with a stable ground throughout this project. August, you were born while I was revising the manuscript. With love and affection, this book is dedicated to all four of you.

I

# Invisibility and Islamic healing in the West

What is it like to be a Muslim who is possessed by a jinn spirit? How do you find refuge from madness and evil spirits when you live in a place like Denmark? In this book I analyse some of the ways in which Muslims in the West have sought to protect themselves. During fieldwork conducted over several years, I followed Muslim patients while they were being treated in a Danish mosque and in a psychiatric hospital. Some of the Muslims I worked with found healing in psychotropic therapy, but many turned to Islam to find protection from the jinn as well as from intrusions by secular state institutions.

My intention has been to specifically explore the role of the invisible in their experiences of mental illness and spirit possession, and as such, this book belongs to a long tradition of studies aiming to understand the invisible in human life. Illnesses such as psychosis and possession occupy an ambiguous position in the borderland between the visible and invisible. Such illnesses are sometimes expressed through visible signs, but the cause of illness and the experience of suffering are often invisible.

Psychiatric healthcare and Islamic exorcism offer different ways of giving the invisible a recognisable shape. Yet both psychiatric healthcare and Islamic exorcism also operate through a disruption of the immediately visible, thereby intensifying the experience of uncertainty and invisibility, of being powerless and in need of help. Both psychiatric healthcare and Islamic exorcism rely on a dissolution of human perceptual agency in favour of submission to external and essentially invisible healing agents – namely, psychotropic medicine and God. In this way, psychiatric treatment and Islamic exorcism raise questions about the limits of human perception and the human capacity for healing.

Readers familiar to Arabic may find the use of the concept of exorcism to be peculiar. In Arabic, the term the people I worked with would use is *al-ruqya al-shar'iyya* – lawful incantation – the common practice of reciting prayers and Quranic verses for healing and protection not only from jinn, but from all kinds of maladies ranging from headaches to severe illness. In analysing a maraboutic approach to the expelling of jinn, Mohammed Maarouf (2007) prefers the concept 'eviction' to avoid the projection of Western ideas of evil on Muslim practices of healing. In a recent book on *ruqya* in Morocco, Stefania Pandolfo (2018: 265–6) also avoids the concept of exorcism to stress that the Quranic cure never completely eliminates the jinn since its harmful invisible power in complex ways 'is internal to the human soul'.

For the people I worked with, the struggle with the jinn is also an ongoing and difficult endeavour. Yet they insist that ultimately the jinn has no business in a human body, and if it is discovered they will do their best to get rid of it. In using the term exorcism (in Danish *eksorcisme* or *åndeud-drivelse*), I am relying on my interlocutors' own efforts to translate and explain their practices, which they recognise as being different from, yet also having important commonalities with, other traditions of exorcism and a common origin in the healing practices shared by both Judaism, Christianity, and Islam (see also Philips 2007). The adoption of the concept of exorcism among many Muslims in Europe as a description of the cures of the jinn could quickly be explained as an effect of Westernisation. Yet it can also be understood as a way of situating the Quranic cures in dialogue with other traditions and as an identification of certain similarities that warrants the use of a common term. One ambition of the project has been to understand how the people I worked with perceive the differences and commonalities of their approaches to healing in relation to other traditions.

My analysis of the invisible in Islamic exorcism and Danish psychiatry comprises both this written commentary and a film. The results take the form of a *film monograph* (Connor, Asch, and Asch 1986). With a camera in hand I have used film as a means to approach the invisible in ways that differ from what has been standard in much writing within the social sciences. In addition I have used the particular sensibilities of the camera as an analytical tool in the theorisation of ritual and healing. Like healing, the production of film can be understood as a practice that despite its visible form essentially has invisible aspects of human life as its principal object (such as experiential and emotional developments within subjects). The aesthetic techniques of both healing and filmmaking can be understood as a sustained process of image-making and image-breaking. Between the cracks of these images the invisible may emerge as an externality beyond the reach of perception. Inspired by theories of cinematic montage, the book and film explore how disruptive techniques are used in healing to destabilise individual perceptions and experiences of agency, so as to allow patients to submit to external powers beyond their own control.

The idea for the project came from previous fieldwork in Kafrat al-Gabal, a suburb of Giza, Egypt, in 2004–5 (Suhr and Bahnsen 2005). While studying sales strategies among camel-drivers at the Pyramids plateau, I lived in the house of a local family of three brothers, their wives, children, and parents. Shortly after my arrival, the wife of the newly wedded youngest brother became possessed by one of the invisible spirits called jinn. Several months proceeded with numerous attempts to cure the woman by way of Quranic recitation, exorcism, prayer, and ritual purification with holy water and honey. I tried hard to convince the family that we should go to a psychiatrist, and also offered to pay for such a consultation as I was increasingly disturbed by the young woman's outbreaks of highly transgressive behaviour, severe fevers, and incomprehensible utterances. While a part of me persistently rejected spirit possession as a proper explanation, I could not help but begin to protect myself from these malicious forces with small home-made supplications to a God I had never and did not want to believe in. Having been raised in the Danish countryside with a good deal of religious scepticism, I felt uncomfortable experiencing how suddenly invisible spiritual forces, evil eyes, and magic slipped into my world.

Driven by a combination of disbelief and curiosity I decided to apply for a scholarship in order to explore the role that such invisible entities could play in the lives of the Muslims in my hometown of Aarhus, Denmark. My fieldwork for this book was slowly initiated in and around the mosques of Aarhus in March 2009 and has continued with several prolonged breaks until the present day. The most important part of the research, including the recording of more than 100 hours of film footage, intensive participant observation, and hundreds of conversations and interviews was carried out in collaboration with people from the mosques between April 2010 and October 2011.

My reasons for moving the project from Egypt to Denmark were primarily practical. As the father of young children, it was more convenient to do long-term fieldwork closer to home. Yet in Denmark new challenges, complexities, and fields of invisibility began to open up. Many of the Islamic healers and Muslim patients I met had personal experiences of or strong opinions about the Danish welfare system, and especially Danish psychiatric healthcare. Indeed the psychiatric system was a primary reference point through which the benefits and dangers of Islamic exorcisms were evaluated. I decided to extend my fieldwork to take a closer look at how Muslim patients experienced the psychiatric system, and to explore the ways in which psychiatrists and nurses dealt with this particular group of patients. Most of my observations of psychiatric consultations occurred between February and October 2011, when I was following the work of psychiatric nurses at the Team for Transcultural Psychiatry and Centre South at Aarhus University Hospital in Risskov.

Having spent months among Islamic healers in the mosques, encountering the psychiatric system quickly became just as unsettling and exotic as my initial encounter with jinn possession years earlier in Egypt. Psychiatric diagnoses and methods of treatment I had previously taken for granted as self-evident truths proven by science now appeared strange and unfamiliar. Jinn possession and paranoid schizophrenia had become equally effective ways of evoking the limits of the visible and knowable within my horizon of experience. This book and the accompanying film explores the ways that Muslim healers, patients, nurses, and psychiatrists experience and understand the healing practices they engage in, and provides the story of my encounters with the invisible in the psychiatric institutions and mosques of Aarhus.

## The invisible in social science and Islam

Intellectual life has for a long time been obsessed with the invisible. Whether defined in terms of actual vision or in the form of hidden ideological, economic, psychological, magical, or religious structures, the invisible has often, as Bruno Latour (1993: 38) points out, been regarded as that which is waiting to be uncovered and made visible. Karl Marx and Friedrich Engels (1988[1844]) proclaimed that the invisible was to be found and exposed in the social processes occurring 'behind the backs' of individual agents. According to Sigmund Freud (1980[1899]), the invisible forces governing our lives could also be discovered in unfulfilled desires hidden within the 'unconscious' of the human psyche. In structuralist anthropology, the invisible was located in universal structures existing before and beyond the individual, directing the tangible form of various social phenomena from kinship alliances and myths to ways of carving a stone (Lévi-Strauss 2001[1978]).

All of these grand social theories revealed that 'facts' are not inscribed on the faces of the objects we encounter, but lie beyond the visible world. Often the ambition of social science has been to provide people with an enlightened vision to liberate them from the invisible forces governing their lives, as in the Marxist struggle to expose 'false consciousness' or in the attempt of psychoanalysis to uncover the 'unconscious'. However, efforts of this sort risk eradicating the essence of the invisible by substituting it with the visibility of pre-established ideas and theories of what it contains.

For the people I worked with in the mosques of Aarhus, belief in the idea that something exists that cannot be seen and cannot be made visible, and that human life is predicated upon such an absolute impermeable invisibility, is a matter of great urgency. Shaykh Abu Bilal who came to Denmark as a Palestinian refugee from Lebanon and later became the imam of the Muslim Society for Equality and Brotherhood in Aarhus, explained the importance of the invisible with an anecdote:

'Once there was a teacher who didn't believe in anything. One day he came to the class and started to ask his students some questions. He asked, "Can you see this chair?" The students answered, "Yes, we see the chair." The teacher said, "This means that now the chair is here. Do you see the blackboard?" The students answered, "Yes." The teacher said, "This means that the blackboard is here." Then he asked, "Can you see God?" "No," the students replied. The teacher concluded, "This means that there is no God." Then a clever child asked the teacher, "Do you think?" "Yes," the teacher answered. The child asked, "Have you learned?" "Yes," he replied. Finally the child asked, "Have you seen your brain?" The teacher said, "No." "So then you don't have a brain," the student concluded.'

For Abu Bilal this short anecdote explains something about the stupidity of our immediate common-sense perception and of purely empiricist science:

'The problem for us today is that everyone wants to see everything. This is because we have been raised on Earth with seeing. But if I went back fifty years in time and said to you that one day they'll produce a mobile phone with which you can call the US, you can see your friends, you can see all kinds of images on the internet, you will say, "No, this is impossible." But now you have this mobile phone. People have produced it. But what about God who has created these people?'

Islam, for Abu Bilal, provides a message about the invisible and guidance for how to believe in it. Yet he emphasises that since the invisible is invisible, it cannot be seen by a human being. To some extent it can be approached through imagination, but it can never be grasped or contemplated as such. Rather than laying bare or somehow offering a map of the invisible, the divine message for Abu Bilal provides a testimony of the enigmatic fact that the invisible is there, beyond the scope of our gaze.

I sometimes asked Abu Bilal why God did not just make everything visible to us. This way life might have been simpler and easier. In Abu Bilal's view, the answer is simple: if the invisible was visible to us, there would be no meaning to the divine test. Everyone would obviously choose paradise over hell. But by disguising hell as a paradise, and by making the other world invisible, God instituted the great test of humankind.

'So why did God do this?' I would ask.

For Abu Bilal continuing this line of enquiry is both impossible and not the point: 'We cannot know the answers to such questions. It would never be possible for us to understand the choices and intentions of God.' The task for humankind is to accept the test that has been given, not to speculate on why it was given.

For Abu Bilal, human life is predicated upon a beyond which lies outside the domain of human perception, power, and knowledge – a beyond which in Islamic theology is encapsulated by the concept of *al-ghayb* (Quran 2: 3, 3: 179, 27: 65; see also Drieskens 2008: 107; Mittermaier 2011: 47; Bubandt, Rytter, and Suhr 2017; Pandolfo 2018). The etymological meaning of *ghayb* comes from the root *gh-ā-ba*, which refers to that which is covered by something else – the unapparent and hidden, that which has gone away, is uncertain, unexposed, and not 'as it seems'. The opposite of *gh-ā-ba* is *sha-hi-da*, referring to the apparent, certain, and immediately visible, that which is exposed and 'as it seems'.

For my interlocutors the dominion of the unseen (*'ālam al-ghayb*) includes not only those parts of visible reality that cannot be seen simply because they are covered or hidden by other visible objects – i.e. that which lies behind this door, or that wall. More important are the kinds of invisibility that cannot by definition be perceived, such as the face or throne of God, paradise, hell, the past, or the future. To act in this world as if the invisible could be seen is the epitome of pious practice. Thus at the deep level of Islamic practice called *iḥsān*, *al-ghayb* has become as integral to the worshipper's perceptual horizon as the immediately visible.

In discussing these issues, Abu Bilal would highlight the story of Abraham – the 'father of faith' in Judaism, Christianity, and Islam. For Abu Bilal the near-sacrifice of Abraham's son at the Mountain of Moriah is one such instance where both son and father succeeded in seeing not the invisible, but the limits of their perception, knowledge, and capacity for judgement in the face of the vastness of the divine plan. When Abraham was asked to sacrifice his son he did not ask why he should do this – rather, he had faith that this was what he was required to do (Quran 37: 102–11; Genesis 22).

It was fascinating for me to hear the shaykh's interpretation of this primal scene of religious sacrifice. In public school I had been brought up with the writings of the Danish philosopher Søren Kierkegaard, for whom Abraham's sacrifice was equally central. As also argued by Kierkegaard (2005[1843]: 38ff), what seems absurd or meaningful within this earthly world may not be so when seen from the viewpoint of a divine being. Both Abu Bilal and Kierkegaard appear to share the view that faith or pious practice is facilitated by the existence of an unknown and infinite invisible without which devotion as an active submission of consciousness would be impossible. Religious belief in this sense is not so much about epistemic certainty as a piece of knowledge one could have or somehow own; rather, it is an act of trust – a submission of one's perception and capacity for action to the supreme ruling of God (see also Schielke 2010: 4; 2019; Luhrmann 2012b: xxi; Willerslev and Suhr 2018).

I should make clear at this stage that the definition of *al-ghayb* asserted by Abu Bilal is characteristic of current neo-orthodox movements of Islam sometimes identified as 'Salafism' or 'Islamic fundamentalism'. These movements can be briefly defined as a striving to achieve what is regarded as a more original, truer practice of faith – namely the practices identified with the immediate companions of the Prophet Muhammad, *al-salaf* (the predecessors; see Sedgwick 2010). Most of my interlocutors would simply describe these practices as the only true embodiment of Islam, and thus do not see themselves as a special branch of Muslims. It is mainly when having to distinguish themselves from what they describe as more 'moderate', 'modern', or 'corrupted' schools of Islamic thought that references to Salafism will be made. Only one person I spoke to explicitly described himself as 'the last Salafi in Aarhus'. All the others were, for him, more or less corrupted 'Sufis'.

In academic writing, concepts such as 'reformist' and 'revivalist' Islam have grown popular (Esposito 1998; Mahmood 2005: 58; Mittermaier 2011: 34). Here I use the term 'neo-orthodox' to avoid any valuation or judgement as to whether Islam in these current movements is literally being 'reformed' or 'revived' or whether it is in fact a matter of Muslims attempting to return to a more original and authentic state of pious practice. The latter would be the position of my interlocutors. For them Islam cannot be reformed, revived, or changed. Rather, it is given to humankind by God as an eternal and universally valid set of directions that lead towards the 'straight path' (*al-ṣirāṭ al-mustaqīm*, Quran 1:6).

Abu Bilal and the other mosque participants place enormous emphasis on a literal interpretation of the Quran as a total system for the conduct of their lives. But since it is impossible for any human being to contain the full meaning of the divine words, Islam leaves considerable room for divergent interpretations. The world of angels, jinn, the prophets, and God, as the endpoint of the 'straight path', is always infinitely deferred into the realm of the invisible.

This understanding of the invisible is not necessarily a view shared by all Muslims. As reported by Amira Mittermaier (2011) in a study of dream-visions in Cairo, Islamic Sufism offers a number of techniques for enhancing the ability to actually see the invisible. As Mittermaier (2011: 89) writes: 'The Prophet, his companions, the angels, and the saints are visible to some but not to others.' According to Mittermaier's interlocutors, invisibility is not a condition accruing to all human beings, but rather an early evolutionary state of perceptual consciousness from which the faithful should try to work their way out. Much disapproval was expressed by my interlocutors over such curious 'Sufi' claims as having 'seen' the Prophet, long-deceased saints, future events, or invisible spirits.

For the people I worked with, the Quranic statement that God is *ghayb* means that in this life God is impossible to see. Yet ideally one should still act in this world as if all that one did see was God. One of the ways in which such a perceptual sensitivity can be cultivated is by remembering that while God is invisible, all that which is visible is ultimately the result of God. As I describe in further details throughout this book, the angels, as well as the invisible spirits called jinn, are also *ghayb,* and for this reason their true form is impossible to see for a human being. Yet both angels and jinn might still be seen when assuming an earthly form. Thus jinn are commonly seen in the shape of a black cat, a snake, or a dog. Likewise the Quran reports how angels took on a human form when addressing the Prophet Muhammad, Abraham, and Lot.

In addition, the presence of angels may be felt while witnessing certain natural phenomena. Abu Bilal and other interlocutors pointed out how – like all blessings, healings, punishments, and illnesses – even the tiniest drops of rain are brought down by angels to the world of humans. While remaining beyond perceptual grasp, the invisible is recognised as effectuating a change in the visible environment which can be seen, and which therefore can be contemplated as an object for the cultivation of a pious perceptual disposition (see also Mittermaier 2011: 24).[1]

Taking the cue from the theories of Abu Bilal and other neo-orthodox Muslims, the invisible in this book is defined in the broadest possible way as that which cannot be directly perceived – at least not from the perspective of a human being. As Charles Hirschkind (2006: 8) has pointed out, the moral vision facilitated by *al-ghayb* is cultivated in important ways through senses other than vision – most notably by listening to recitations of the divine words of the Quran. Yet it is clear that even though messages from *al-ghayb* can be communicated through sound, the dominion of the unseen cannot be grasped completely through hearing or any other sense. Nor is the invisible just a metaphor for the unknown – rather, it is precisely that which cannot be known. In short the invisible, as used here, is that which entirely exceeds our human faculties of perception and knowledge.

## The invisible as invisible

The similarity between Kierkegaard and Abu Bilal's interpretations of Abraham's sacrifice is one of several interesting resemblances between the Islamic notion of *al-ghayb* and the understanding of the invisible in certain strands of existential, phenomenological, and ethical philosophy. These philosophies allow us to further develop a concept of invisibility in relation to our perception of the things that surround us, as well as the invisible within ourselves. In an age where Islam and the West are increasingly defined as antagonistic opposites, there are complexities – but also much relevance – in acknowledging the similarities of thinking in both Muslim and Western philosophy (see also Marks 2010 and Sedgwick 2016). Throughout the book I return to these philosophies when analysing the differences and similarities of psychiatric healthcare and Islamic exorcism.

In Maurice Merleau-Ponty's (2002[1945]) phenomenology of perception, the invisible is described as an implication and a necessary part of all human perception. Indeed, it is a condition for perception. Merleau-Ponty explores this hypothesis at the level of motor-intentional actions. When trying, for example, to grip this cup at the table, my hand intuits where to place the tips of the fingers, as if the fingertips had seen the back of the cup before ever travelling the distance from the front of the cup to its other side. In some way I, my body, and my fingertips intuit the invisible terrain of the back of the cup before actually seeing it. In Merleau-Ponty's understanding, this is because the actual perspective of any human being always already presupposes the vast network of alternative perspectives that lie behind the cup and make up its invisible side. I see the cup sitting on the table as a fully-fledged three-dimensional object because the actual visual perspective of my eyes automatically and intuitively takes into account all other possible positions from where I could have seen the cup, but which from my present perspective are invisible (see also Merleau-Ponty 1997[1964]; Kelly 2005; Suhr and Willerslev 2012).

As pointed out by Elisabetta Basso (2011: 242), perception in the sense described by Merleau-Ponty is a form of faith – a trust in our relatedness to the world – a gesture of certitude that operates despite the fact that the things surrounding us are never completely visible. Indeed this expression of faith operating at the level of our motor-intentional actions is not so different from the form of faith and certitude (*tawakkul*, *yaqīn*) described by both Abu Bilal and Kierkegaard in their analysis of the story of Abraham and his son (see also Basso 2011: 249). To paraphrase Kierkegaard, Merleau-Ponty's phenomenology of perception is a paradoxical perception, which works only on the strength of that which cannot be directly perceived.

Inspired by gestalt theory, Merleau-Ponty (1964[1948]: 49; see also Kelly 2005: 91) declares that all human vision is guided by a 'norm'. The infinite totality of possible viewpoints surrounding us and surrounding the objects of our gaze provides the invisible ground upon which objects present themselves as visible. This 'total invisible' or infinite 'view from everywhere' – that is, the universe as seen from all sides, at all times, all at once – is for Merleau-Ponty the condition and the guiding ideal for human perception. This panoptic viewpoint – *al-Baṣīr*, God as the All-Seeing, as it would be called in Islamic theology – though unreachable from any human perspective, operates, according to Merleau-Ponty (2002: 79, 352), as an invisible norm that provides the necessary ground for any perspectival seeing.

In recent years a number of anthropologists and theoreticians have been inspired by Merleau-Ponty's theory of object perception (Holenstein 1999; Kelly 2005; Holbraad and Willerslev 2007: 335; Pedersen 2011). In a sense these authors appear to be putting us back inside the cave so famously described by Plato. Yet in Merleau-Ponty, as Rane Willerslev (2009a: 33) makes clear, there is no going outside the cave and no possible ascent to full panoptic seeing. To be human means to be embodied in the particular, enmeshed and chained in the matrix of the visible, hence only having partial, indirect access to the total invisible. Objectivity in such a theory of object perception is decidedly not about being able to fully grasp an object, but instead quite the opposite. An object becomes visible to us only when it is partly invisible, that is, when we recognise that there is a hidden side which we cannot perceive from our present position (Kelly 2005: 78; see also Haraway 1991).

For our purposes here, we may note the resemblance between neo-orthodox Islamic notions of invisibility and truth and the theory of objectivity proposed by Merleau-Ponty. Wherever we direct our gaze and stare at the visible facades of the world, both Merleau-Ponty and neo-orthodox Islam teach us how the invisible sneaks along, hiding in the shadows behind and between, at the periphery, or even within the objects of our gaze. Although we cannot see it, and regardless of whether or not we choose to admit its presence, the invisible is somehow always with us. Yet for my interlocutors, appreciation of the invisible origin of the visible is not just a matter of correct perception. In important ways, it is connected to ethics.

## The invisible face of the Other

When looking at one another, we quickly find ourselves in the realm of the invisible. Something is occurring within you as we face each other. I sense this, although I cannot see it. For Emmanuel Levinas (1985) this is the experience of encountering the invisible face of the Other. This invisible face hides beneath the facial expression of the other. For Levinas, it conveys an uncontrollable, inaccessible, and irreducible 'excess of otherness', which can never be seen or adequately portrayed (Wyschogrod 2002: 191). The invisible, therefore, is not simply the result of incomplete perception or knowledge. According to Levinas: 'Invisibility results … from the inaptitude of knowledge as such – from its inadequation – to the infinity of the absolutely other' (1987a: 32; see also Merleau-Ponty 1976; Basso 2011: 253). It is in this sense that the face of the other 'is not seen' and cannot be captured within thought. Rather, the face is alterity beyond representation. It is the 'uncontainable' – that which 'leads you beyond' (Levinas 1985: 86–7).

For Levinas, it is not the case that the other needs protection from attempts to reduce its otherness to any recognisable representation. Rather, the perceiving self is conditioned upon its relation to the other and therefore must embrace the other's irreducible and infinite otherness. The vulnerable and powerless condition of the self in the face of the other is made clear by Levinas in his description of the impossibility of murdering alterity: 'The Other, whose exceptional presence is inscribed in the ethical impossibility of killing him in which I stand, marks the end of powers. If I can no longer have power over him it is because he overflows absolutely every idea I can have of him' (Levinas 1979[1961]: 87).

Despite their theoretical differences, both Levinas's notion of invisibility as the irreducible 'face of the other' and Merleau-Ponty's ever-present 'view from everywhere' bear a close affinity to Kierkegaard's concept of the 'absolute' and 'infinite', as well as the concept of God as expressed among my neo-orthodox Muslim interlocutors. All of these concepts refer to a form of unreachable normative ideal – a plenitude of perspectives that we cannot do without. It underlies every perspective as the invisible background that allows things to stand out in their visibility. Yet it must hide itself in order for the visible world to appear before our eyes. As Merleau-Ponty (2000: 187) articulates: 'the proper essence ... of the visible is to have a layer of invisibility ... which it makes present by a certain absence.' As such, the 'view from everywhere' and 'the other' cannot be an object of our own subjective seeing except negatively, that is, through its absence.

But we need not even go out into the world or find other human beings in order to encounter the invisible. As Jean-Paul Sartre (2000[1943]: 260) observed, that which we cannot see by our own power, is also our own seeing. When looking directly at ourselves in a mirror we find the invisible staring back at us from the dark spaces in the midst of our eyes. What hides there?

When writing this book, I sometimes asked, 'who is it who thinks and writes this sentence?' Instead of finding a 'cogito', such as that described by René Descartes, a slightly disturbing experience took place. Under close examination, cogito often loses its familiarity. Not by necessity does any unification in the shape of an 'I' occur. Who is it who thinks and writes this sentence? When asking myself this question, cloudy shadows begin to move, disappear, reappear, and disappear again. For me, an overwhelming experience of not being alone and of finding not cogito but rather multiple 'someones/somethings' quickly ends this line of speculation.

According to studies on psychosis and schizophrenia in cognitive psychology, such an experienced lack of cogito is not as alarming as it might appear. Indeed, as pointed out by Chris Harrop and Peter Trower (2003: 67–8), Descartes himself might have been suffering from a psychological malfunction, since full identification between perceiving 'I' and perceived 'me' can be characteristic of emerging schizophrenia. This is the self in which the invisible has been entirely eradicated, replaced by a blind faith in the idea that ego equals ego and that the world is as it appears (see also Deleuze 2005b[1989]: 129). Hence, for example, the horror of the psychiatric patient who found himself in full faith that 'Yes, this is me, I am Stalin'. This is the self characterised by a destructive combination of 'egocentricity, idealism, and black/white thinking' (Harrop 2002: 296). By contrast, the experience of not being entirely alone within one's own body and mind should, as asserted by Harrop and Trower (2003: 187), not automatically be regarded as a symptom of psychosis. As affirmed by studies of voice-hearing, it is not necessarily pathological that an 'I' often experiences its interior world as including multiple invisible 'others' (Romme and Escher 2000; Nielsen,

Mikkelsen, and Aagaard 2009; Luhrmann 2012a). Rather, it is a relatively 'normal', and sometimes even necessary, experience.

This brief Cartesian meditation is just one particular encounter with the invisible. The long tradition of invisibility studies offers many different attempts to understand how the confrontation between humankind and the invisible takes on particular forms and meanings in diverse cultural and social contexts. This book is one such study of the invisible in human life. It is situated in a historical and cultural setting where the invisible takes forms that need not be generalisable on a universal scale. Yet the study is predicated upon the general hypothesis that since the invisible is invisible, no human being can come to see it or know it exactly as it is.

## Invisibility in Denmark

My fieldwork was conducted among psychiatrists, nurses, shaykhs, and Muslim patients in Denmark. Even in such a limited geographical context, the invisible appears too broad a concept for an anthropological investigation. One way of further delineating a study of the invisible is to look at what people do when they encounter the invisible. In the Danish context, several types of response may be observed.

Sometimes people appear to embrace the invisible in its invisibility, without attempting to render it visible but by accepting its invisibility and dealing with it as such. This, it seems, is the way Levinas, Merleau-Ponty, and also Kierkegaard would have it. In their terms this would not only be ethically correct but also a logical response, since not to acknowledge the existence of the invisible would be to disable one's capacity for proper perception and action.

More frequently, however, people would try to ignore the invisible and attempt to go about their business as if the invisible was not there. Denial or indifference here becomes the modality through which the invisible is encountered.

At other times, the encounter may evoke within people the desire to make visible, to attack, or even to conquer the invisible, a response which would sit at the other end of Levinas's and Merleau-Ponty's scale. As Levinas points out, making otherness and the invisible visible is the opposite of ethics – it is the basic violation of otherness. A violation that not only denies otherness but leads to the destruction of the self, since the self cannot subsist without the other.

When I conducted my fieldwork it could – on the surface of things – appear as if many Danes did not particularly like the invisible. As in other places around the world, the invisible is sometimes connected to darkness, and even to danger (Bille and Sørensen 2007: 272; Vigh and Turner 2007:

7). Denmark, as a Northern European country, has a strong history of Protestantism and certain ideals inherited from the Enlightenment. Danes have even been characterised as devotees of a radical form of 'normative secularism' – a movement or school of thought which holds that 'rational', 'informed', and 'enlightened' thought should govern, and that 'religious', 'irrational', and 'spiritual' behaviour should be strictly confined to the private sphere of individuals.[2] However, at the same time the teaching of Christianity (*kristendomskundskab*) is mandatory in Danish public schools and the Danish state also sponsors an official Protestant state church, the *folkekirken* (Sedgwick 2014). Every Sunday morning church bells can be heard across the country. Nevertheless, explicit expressions of firm and unconditional faith in a transcendent invisible truth have almost acquired the status of blasphemy.

This was seen when, in 2013, the congregation of a Danish village church straightforwardly advertised a vacant position for 'a priest who believed in God' (Politiken 2013). The reaction of the chairman of the Danish Society of Priests, Per Bucholdt Andreasen, was prompt: 'This is getting close to mind control [*sindelagskontrol*].' The former Minister for Gender Equality and Ecclesiastical Affairs, Manu Sareen, was equally disturbed and said he hoped 'this was a formulation that the congregation had not properly thought through'.

As in much social science, the invisible is often regarded as something which ought to be made visible, illuminated, uncovered, and mapped so that conscious, rational thought can place it under control and act on it (Sjørslev 2002: 30; Vigh and Turner 2007; Vacher 2010; Larsen 2011). Danes seem to treasure openness, transparency, and exact knowledge, to the extent that they have become one of the most monitored, counted, registered, catalogued, and statistically enumerated populations in the world (Lauritsen 2011). Every citizen has a special number that directly links them to a precise individual trajectory from birth, through kindergarten, education, work, marriage, reproduction, hospitalisation, dental records, court cases, real estate investments, death, etc. On account of these statistics Denmark has for a number of years been identified as the least corrupt and most transparent country in the world (Transparency International 2016). Also on account of these statistics and additional surveys – but in spite of somewhat negative employment, mental health, and suicide records – researchers have continuously claimed that Danes are in fact among the happiest populations in the world, only competing for the prestigious title with countries such as Finland, Norway, and Switzerland (Helliwell, Layard, and Sachs 2012, 2016, 2019; see also White 2006).

However, certain parts of the country and certain parts of the population are usually not mentioned in this rhetoric of transparency, happiness, and visibility. In public discourse some of these places are officially referred to as the 'ghettos'. These places and their inhabitants are often invisible in the appraisals of Denmark as a country of happiness and transparency, yet they become hypervisible when politicians and commentators attempt to locate the causes of negative employment and mental health records as well as the relatively large amount of the Danish population receiving incapacity benefits (Jeldoft 2013; Rytter and Pedersen 2014; Johansen and Jensen 2017).

The Danish government has defined a 'ghetto' as a social housing complex whose inhabitants consists of more than 50 per cent immigrants or descendants of immigrants from non-Western countries. Furthermore a 'ghetto' is defined by having an unemployment rate among its inhabitants of at least 40 per cent as well as a higher than average ratio of crime.[3]

The 'ghetto' where most of the fieldwork for this study was carried out is known as Gellerupparken and Toveshøj. Since beginning my research, the number of inhabitants has decreased from more than 7,000 to 6,000 people. Currently 81 per cent are registered as 'immigrants or descendants of immigrants from non-Western countries', mainly from Palestine, Lebanon, Somalia, and Turkey. 52 per cent of the inhabitants between 18 and 64 are not active in the labour market, and most of these receive welfare payments. 15 per cent receive student allowances. The remaining 33 per cent are registered either as employed or temporarily unemployed.[4]

In some ways the 'ghetto' seems to meet rational, modern, secular, enlightened ideals of practical planning brilliantly. The large modernist housing complex dominated by tall buildings with square, equally-sized apartments, balconies, and parking lots seem to suggest nothing other than precisely this emphasis on the abstract, timeless equality between individuals within a bounded space that has been taken as an emblem of the modern, secular nation state (Anderson 1991; Scott 1998). Yet like most other 'ghettos', Gellerupparken seems a world apart from the rest of Denmark.

Certainly many of the inhabitants of the areas designated as 'ghettos' are noticeably darker than the stereotypical white, blonde Dane. Most of them speak Danish but with an accent – variously referred to as 'perkerdansk' (derogatory wordplay on Persian-Danish), 'araberslang' (Arab slang), 'grilldansk', or 'multi-ethnolect' (Quist 2000; Christensen 2003).

The Danish media is saturated with stories of young people from these areas who reportedly get into trouble at school or discos, with gangs in the streets, and sometimes end up as problematic records in the unemployment and crime statistics (Ministry of Social Affairs 2011). Some statisticians have argued that the media and politicians heavily overdramatise the difference between what – in an attempt to avoid racialised categories – has become verbalised as 'old' and 'new' Danes; the latter category referring to refugees from non-Western countries and so-called 'guest workers' (*gæstearbejdere*) who came to Denmark from Turkey in the 1960s and 1970s, their children, and their children's children, most of whom have obtained citizenship.

While unemployment rates and illiteracy are often high among first-generation immigrants who came to Denmark as refugees from non-Western countries, their children are catching up at impressive speed, falling behind their so-called 'ethnic' Danish peers by only a few points, and in effect constituting a social leap that would be hard to imagine for 'ethnic' Danish children of similar social and economic backgrounds (Borberg 2016; Rytter 2018).[5] The great attention that the 'ghetto' of Gellerupparken receives as a place that links unemployment and crime with a high number of immigrants also obscures that 80 per cent of immigrants or descendants of immigrants from non-Western countries in the Aarhus Municipality live outside these areas and perform significantly better in employment and crime statistics. Nevertheless most politicians and the Danish media continue to focus on the fact that despite their significant progress, immigrants from non-Western countries and their descendants still perform slightly worse than average.

A similar focus is found when authorities consider the physical and mental health statistics of immigrants and descendants of immigrants (Ringgaard 2012). The Danish Research Centre for Transcultural Psychiatry advocates a degree of caution, however, since health statistics do not always properly distinguish between different categories of immigrants. Yet psychiatrists have found that those who count as so-called 'transcultural patients' – i.e. are immigrants or descendants of immigrants from non-Western countries – do seem to have a significantly higher risk of developing psychotic, affective, and neurotic disorders (Videnscenter for Transkulturel Psykiatri 2012; see also Helweg-Larsen et al. 2007; Norredam et al. 2009). Some scholars have criticised the use of categories such as 'transcultural patients' or 'patients with a non-Danish ethnic background' pointing to the potential risk of automatically equating perceived difference with psychiatric conditions of a special kind (Johansen 2007; see also Foucault 1988[1961]; Hacking 1999). Yet most scholars agree that there are problems that are specific to this part of the population which demand particular attention.

Most scholars and some politicians explain the various issues categorised collectively as 'integration problems' by referring to the traumatic experiences of many first-generation immigrants as a result of fleeing from conflict in the Middle East, and the discrimination and exclusion of immigrants and their children in the educational system and the Danish labour market. But one additional factor not included in the statistics, and which is therefore still partly invisible to the system, is that of religion (Kühle 2006: 38; Jacobsen 2007, 2008). Since the 1990s Danish politicians and opinion makers have increasingly claimed that Islam is in fact the real underlying obstacle to the integration of non-Western immigrants into Danish society (see Hervik 2011; Rytter 2018).

## Is Islam the invisible cause of 'integration problems'?

Walking around in the 'ghetto' of Gellerupparken, it is clearly visible that many of the inhabitants do not conform to the way religion in Denmark is usually laid out to be a strictly private matter. In Gellerupparken religion is something you can physically embody and display in your dress and in the length of your beard. Here you will see men with full beards in calf-length tunics, women wearing headscarves, even a few covered entirely by black robes, despite the fact that the *niqāb* has recently been made illegal by law. Such scarves, beards, and tunics are unmistakably visible signs that these people are practising Muslims.

As Mikkel Rytter (2010a) has pointed out in a study of the ethno-nationalism conjured by the notion of 'family Denmark', people who visually display religious devotion in such ways are not considered to exhibit the 'national attachment' required of 'real Danes'. Among several examples Rytter (2010a: 303) analyses the statements of the former Minister of Education, Integration, Health, Culture, and the Church, Bertel Haarder, who claimed that such people 'live in a subculture outside the Danish tribe' (see also Larsen 2011; and see Fernando 2010 for an analysis of the situation in France).

While Islam may be highly visible in the 'ghettos', it is not immediately visible anywhere else in the otherwise extensive statistics of the Danish population, except if one considers ethnic categories as a marker of religious faith. Since religion is formally considered a private matter, it is simply not legal to produce statistics based directly on people's religion (Kühle 2006: 38). Arguing against the extreme overstatements of right wing politicians as well as acknowledged political scientists, Brian Arly Jacobsen (2008: 84) has pointed out the need for more precise methods of calculating the exact number of Muslims, a more accurate definition of who counts as a Muslim, and for differentiating between those who are simply relatives of immigrants from Muslim majority countries and those who actually practise Islam as an integral part of their everyday life.

Leading politicians and commentators in Denmark also share the desire for more transparent, accurate data on the Muslim population – but not for the same reasons as most scholars of Islam. A few years ago a representative of a group of young Salafi Muslims in Denmark declared his hope that all Danish soldiers in Afghanistan would return in coffins: 'They are fighting for a democracy that we do not want' (cited in Jyllandsposten 2011). The reaction of the former Minister of Integration, Karen Hækkerup, was prompt: 'This is disturbing and disgusting ... We shall map these environments.'[6]

In an enlightened, transparent, and democratic state like Denmark, persons who express discontent with democracy, Danish integration policies, and, in this case, discontent with the attempt to eliminate terrorism through warfare, are not merely seen as unacceptable – they are grotesque and incomprehensible, and as such constitute a riddle that has to be solved. The invisible cause needs to be identified and made visible so that the proper treatment can be prescribed.

One recurrent topic in the public debate is the outrage it created among Muslims in Denmark and elsewhere when Danish cartoonists in 2005 attempted to visualise the Prophet Muhammad in a series of cartoons (see also Hervik 2006; Keane 2009; Mahmood 2009; Boe 2017). What could possibly be so provocative about this? Why shouldn't anything be susceptible to being visualised, drawn in caricature, and made fun of? While some scholars problematised the event as an attempt to stigmatise Muslims (Boe and Hervik 2008), the refusal of visualisation appeared mainly to emphasise that Islam does not conform to the norms of a modern, enlightened, rational, and secular society (Stage 2011: 51). For many commentators it looks suspicious when Muslims so insistently try to keep the face of a certain historical person invisible.

As Talal Asad (2003: 160) has argued, the problem many commentators have with Muslim immigrants in Europe is not so much that they come from another culture, but that they believe in Islam. Garbi Schmidt, Birgitte Johansen, and Dorthe Possing (2008: 3) note how scholars who refuse to acknowledge the threat posed by Islam 'are often described as naively portraying Muslims as victims of Western domination'.

Frequently, politicians and public debaters in Denmark have diagnosed Islam as a kind of social illness responsible for the problems of Muslim immigrants and sometimes Danish society itself. This view was expressed on the webpage of former Member of Parliament Louise Frevert, who compared Danish Muslims to the cells of a malignant tumour:

> If the doctor was to heal his patients with something similar to 'integration' it would mean that he should try to convince the cancer cells to become good, well-functioning, healthy cells that could work harmoniously in the body of the patient. … We may spend billions of kroner [Danish currency] and hours trying to integrate Muslims into this country, but the result is what the doctor observes: the cancer expands itself, unhindered, while we talk. (cited in Information 2005; see also Hervik 2011)

Although Louise Frevert was roundly criticised for the statements on her webpage, this line of thought is increasingly found across a wide spectrum of the political landscape. If malignant cells (sometimes also described more specifically as potential 'Islamist terror cells') can be identified as the cause of the spread of such infectious, irrational hatred of democracy, then they are 'matter out of place' which 'must be cleansed or eradicated' (Douglas 2002[1966]; see also Herzfeld 1992: 38). As Member of Parliament Marie Krarup claims: 'We are at war with the Islamic civilization' and 'we don't have a chance against the 3–4 times higher fertility rate from the Middle East and Africa' (cited in Politiken 2012).

In March 2016 a documentary, entitled *The Mosques Behind the Veil* (Thyrri and Jensen), screened primetime over four nights on the national Danish broadcast channel TV2, applied candid cameras and undercover journalists to investigate whether mosques and imams were promoting or hindering the integration of Danish Muslims. The documentary seemingly exposed imams legitimating social fraud, polygamy, forced sex, the beating of women and children, while denying Muslim women's right to divorce, and discouraging interactions between Muslim and non-Muslim Danes. Specifically the journalists aimed to reveal the hypocrisy of imams by making the differences between their official statements and what imams say internally to their co-believers visible to the Danish public.

The documentary received severe criticism from a number of scholars for misrepresenting statements by imams through selective editing, for insinuating social fraud without proper documentation, and for systematically ignoring everything that would suggest more complex explanations than mosques and imams being the primary cause of Danish integration problems (see e.g. Skovgaard-Petersen 2016; Suhr 2016; Vinding 2016). Despite criticism, the documentary laid the ground for an enormous public outcry (364 articles, 76 TV-features) and far-reaching political initiatives – including legislation to limit the freedom of speech and freedom of religion.

Politicians at the highest level of government were clear in their condemnation of mosques and imams, and generous with metaphors of illness and contagion. Former Minister of Education, Integration, Health, Culture, and the Church, Bertel Haarder, warned against 'rabid imams, who are spreading a death cult'. Søren Espersen, Vice-Chairman of the Danish People's Party, labelled so-called 'Islamist' mosques as 'a violence- and death-glorifying cult, a plague over Denmark'. The Prime Minister at the time, Lars Løkke Rasmussen, stated how such imams 'preach their messages of hatred – preach and spread messages which aim at undermining our democracy'. Echoing previous demands from other politicians, a majority in the parliament agreed 'there was a need for an updated mapping of mosques in Denmark' (see Suhr and Sinclair 2016).

As elsewhere in Europe and North America, Danish Muslims have become increasingly invisible as citizens but hypervisible as potential problems and threats. The Muslim communities that I worked with became the subject of intense public attention and state surveillance due to the above-mentioned documentary as well as their criticism of the cartoons of the Prophet in 2005–6 and accusations that they took part in the radicalisation of a number of young Danish Muslims. Through the process of my research I became intensively engaged in these escalating debates (Suhr et al. 2017). A focus of my research has been to understand how these broader social and political issues have parallels in the invisible dynamics of jinn possession and psychosis.

## Illness and invisibility

Quite obviously, Danish Muslims do not readily agree with the characterisation of Islam as an illness or an invisible cause of 'integration problems'. Rather, most of the people I worked with conceive of Islam as a source of guidance in order to face problems and with which to potentially treat physical as well as mental illnesses.

In Arabic, insane can roughly be translated to *majnūn*. The root letters of *majnūn* are *jīm* and *nūn*, indicating a connection to the word jinn, the invisible spirits that keep mainly to their own world but are sometimes reported to enter the world of humankind (Al-Issa 2000: xv).[7] Although the existence of invisible jinn is attested to in the Quran, many Danish Muslims will frequently deny the relevance of their existence to our earthly life. For some Muslims, jinn is a concept of complex theological significance which ordinary people do not need to consider in depth (see also Rytter 2010b: 49). Others hold we should not burden ourselves thinking about the jinn since God himself states in the Quran that a veil has been created to separate the world of humankind from the invisible world of the spirits. For many Muslims, however, jinn play a crucial role in the earthly life of humankind. Often jinn will play games with humans and will even enter into the bodies of women and men, making them do or say things they would never think of themselves. At times jinn will tease people to the extent of driving them insane – *majnūn*. For some Muslims in Denmark, the attacks, the luring, and the whispering of evil jinn are thought to be the real, invisible cause of the relatively low mental health records of the immigrant population (see also Dein, Alexander, and Napier 2008; Dein and Illaiee 2013).

Some of the so-called (and sometimes self-declared) 'fundamentalist/ Islamist/anti-democratic' Muslims see the treatments for mental health problems offered by the Danish welfare state as a disguised attack on the integrity of faithful Muslims; an attack which is also ultimately directed by *shayāṭīn* (evil jinn), whose aim it is to drag the faithful away from the truth and into the eternal flames of hell. Psychiatric medication for what in a Western context would be diagnosed as depression, stress, anxiety, paranoia, bipolar disorder, or schizophrenia is seen by some Muslims as a subtle weapon for use against the spiritual health of the righteous. Psychiatric drugs, they argue, work not primarily to heal, but rather to pacify your consciousness and your emotional and sensorial faculties, and hence remove you further from divine truth.

From this view, the only thing able to maintain a healthy soul is Islam. Such statements as 'a true Muslim can never get depression' and 'medication only makes you sleep' were frequently uttered in the mosques where I worked. These views are by no means shared by all Muslims in Denmark, but when Muslim patients enter a consultation at a Danish psychiatric hospital, these views are often part of the discursive framework through which they attempt to make sense of the treatment. For the patient, the encounter with the healer – whether Muslim or non-Muslim, exorcist or psychiatrist – presents yet another encounter with the invisible. Just as the cause and form of the suffering is invisible, so are the possible paths for its healing. How do you know whether the healer (*al-mu'ālij*) is sent by angels or *shayāṭīn*?

## The agency of the invisible

When observing how people and institutions react when confronted with the invisible, it is not always clear where to situate or how to define human perceptual agency. Is it human beings who are gradually conquering the invisible, or is the invisible luring humans into worlds of apparent clarity and visibility, only to then overwhelm them with even larger, denser, and inaccessible realms of invisibility?

Regardless of the normative theories of philosophers, anthropologists, Muslim shaykhs, psychiatrists, policy makers, and ordinary people, one feature of the invisible is that we cannot do much about it. We may try to turn on the light when entering a dark room, and although certain things are then lit up, other things hiding deeper in the shadows immediately attract our attention. Indeed the light may be seen as intensifying and expanding the invisible.

Drawing a map brings colours and lines to unknown territories – rendering visible to the human eye a formerly impossible world of perception. Yet as James Scott (1998: 7) points out, the map cannot do this without simultaneously evoking that vastly greater space of still unknown territory surrounding the space it makes visible. Looking at neuroimaging, Allan Young (2011) describes how early promises of an almost full visualisation of the cognitive processes of the brain through modern scanning techniques are now giving way to theories about presumed, though invisible and excessively complex, social processes taking place at the level of 'mirror neurons'.

So it is with the 'ghettos' and the so-called 'integration problems' in Denmark. Despite the fact that the 'ghettos' are some of the most monitored, analysed, publicly debated, and hyper-visualised areas in this country, the causes of their problems still lie hidden in the invisible (Rytter and Pedersen 2014). Science and social science as the enterprise of bringing light upon, mapping, scanning, and visualising the invisible is in this sense nothing but an explosion or amplifier of invisibility.

As Latour (1993: 130, 136) points out, what characterises many social scientists educated in the 'modern secular' era is a belief in humans as capable of objectively perceiving and stepping outside of invisible structures and the 'barbarian medley' of past traditions that govern their lives, thereby creating a new world for themselves in their own image. Many anthropological studies concerned with agency, practice, and the pragmatics and phenomenology of healing appear to reiterate this view of human agency as resistance to external, invisible forces. Thus there has been an emphasis on showing how even physically and mentally ill patients, for all their suffering, still have agency, how illnesses such as psychosis or spirit possession might actually be a form of agentive human resistance, and how practices of healing are not only to be seen as attempts to recover from illness, but are in fact the site of alternative forms of self-creation (see e.g. Csordas 1997; see also Boddy 1989 and Callan 2012).

In this study of psychiatry and Islamic exorcism I have become interested in how, despite the apparent obsession with visibility in Denmark, certain forms of invisible, even non-human agency, not dissimilar to the understanding of the invisible in neo-orthodox Islam, appear to be lurking right beneath the surface of public and scholarly discourse. The greatest surprise for me has been the similarities between what I initially thought were two highly distinctive and even incommensurable practices of healing. While making the suffering of patients visible through diagnoses such as depression, schizophrenia, or jinn possession, the practices not only of Muslim healers but also of psychiatrists and nurses seem directed at facilitating a situation where patients can voluntarily submit themselves to the workings of invisible agents such as God and psychotropic medicine. Healing practices, both in the mosques and in psychiatric institutions, prompt us to consider the scope of human perceptual agency as a power of resistance and self-creation, and to also consider if, when, and to what extent such powers are desirable.

In my analysis of Islamic and psychiatric approaches to healing, I have been much inspired by debates in the anthropology of Islam that have in various ways problematised the notion of autonomous, self-possessed human agency (see e.g. Mahmood 2005; Hirschkind 2006; Mittermaier 2011). In her analysis of spiritual dispossession in Morocco, Pandolfo (2018) discusses the agency of images, of traumatic traces, of the jinn, of destruction as such, and, not least, the agency of God as related to the healing practices of Muslim shaykhs. Combining psychoanalysis with Islamic theology, Pandolfo demonstrates how the renewal of life is made possible when patients and healers overcome their fear of illness and embrace death as the ultimate destiny (see also Irving 2017). In several ways the material I discuss here points to the conclusions proposed in Pandolfo's work. In Denmark the idea of humans as free agentive individuals has long been a dominating model both of and for the conduct of social and political life. Here, however, I address the agency of human beings – not as an analytic concept – but rather as a particular existential problem which shaykhs, psychiatrists, nurses, and patients struggle with and seek to overcome.

The basic and perhaps commonplace message suggested by the healing practices of shaykhs, nurses, and psychiatrists is that peace of mind, and the experience of freedom does not always rest in people's ability to act, to throw away tradition and myth, maximise resources, and become masters of life or producers of structure. Sometimes it lies in the ability of persons to submit themselves to a pre-existing structure. This understanding of freedom and agency can also be found in Merleau-Ponty's work on the phenomenology of perception. As he states: 'I can miss being free only if I try to bypass my natural and social situation by refusing to take it up … Nothing determines me from outside, not because nothing acts on me, but, on the contrary, because I am from the start outside myself and open to the world' (Merleau-Ponty 2002: 529–30).

For Claude Lévi-Strauss the ability to join oneself to the structuring powers of an outside is the very locus of human creativity. What Lévi-Strauss (1983[1964]: 12) claimed to show was 'not how men [*sic*] think in myths, but how myths operate in men's [*sic*] minds without their being aware of the fact'. Indeed Lévi-Strauss argued that 'perhaps [it would] be better to go still further and, disregarding the thinking subject completely, proceed as if the thinking process were taking place in the myths, in their reflection upon themselves and their interrelation' (1983[1964]: 12). Recounting the production of his massive corpus of text, the 'father of structuralism' denied that his authorship could be attributed to his own ability to perceive, master, and bring order to the material collected in the field. Instead he saw it as the production of myth by myth or a kind of 'myth of myths'. As he writes:

> It is hard for me to perceive myself as a person, as an I. I am a site where certain things happen in a transitory manner. Thought is like water passing through a sieve that completely escapes me. I can't recuperate memories of my past. I suffer from a total lack of identity … the ethnologist in his office trying to be a place where foreign thoughts develop … this infirmity of my nature makes me almost a passive place since I don't control what happens, almost a passive site of phenomena that don't belong to my own existence, to my own history, or my social milieu. (Lévi-Strauss on his hundredth birthday, quoted in Marcus 2013; see also Willerslev and Suhr 2018)

Lévi-Strauss identified how the structuring invisible power of myth was at work not only among indigenous people in the Amazon, but also deeply embedded within his own work, and in the rational thinking of modern science. Like Lévi-Strauss, I wish with this book to scratch beneath the discursive facades of modern secular thought. Both psychiatric healthcare and Islamic exorcisms suggest a view of healing and human creativity as essentially operating through submission to external, invisible forms of extra-human agency. Thus I aim to show not only how Islamic exorcisms, but equally the modern institution of psychiatry – despite its claims to rational objectivity – are entangled in a variety of ritual practices that have the mythical and, what I broadly conceive of as the invisible, as its principal point of reference.[8]

## Film and the invisible

A particular ambition in my research has been to combine film and text in ways that would enable me to approach invisible phenomena such as jinn, magic, and psychosis, which appear to be so difficult to contain within the logic of a single set of analytic categories. What initially prompted me to go beyond written analysis was quite simply that my experience of these phenomena could not be contained within the descriptive tools I had available. At the beginning of this project I thought that film would somehow allow me a more holistic access to such experiences.

In the sub-discipline of visual anthropology, the value of film has often been located in its capacity to allow us the experience of 'being there' and 'seeing for ourselves'. Lucien Castaing-Taylor (1996: 75–6) emphasises how the long takes of a camera honour the duration of real-life interaction and 'the homogeneity of space by preserving the relationships between objects'. In a similar vein, Paul Henley (2004: 114) argues that film, as long as it remains undisturbed by excessive aesthetic manipulation, may allow intimate access to the subjective seeing of the camera operator. Both Henley and Castaing-Taylor point out how the constant flow of images, sounds, and words in film parallels the way humans experience reality more closely than any other medium of communication.

While I initially shared this assumption of a correspondence between subjective human perception and the recordings of a camera, gradually I have become more sceptical. A number of anthropologists, theorists, and filmmakers have pointed out how film – while clearly operating in different sensorial and conceptual registers than written text – still reduces lived reality and human experience, no less than textual categories and analytic schemes (see e.g. Arnheim 1957; Trinh 1991; Vaughan 1992; Weiner 1997; Marks 2000). Ethnographic filmmaking, and especially the branch of observational cinema, have been criticised as yet another Enlightenment project of visualising the world – an ocular-centric colonising enterprise that fetishises the camera as a kind of 'audiovisual vacuum cleaner, voraciously sucking in time and space' (Kiener 2008: 405; see also Köhn 2016: 85–6).

To be sure, looking at film is not the same thing as being immersed in pro-filmic reality. Rather than 'being there' and 'seeing for ourselves', film-viewing can sometimes be a disturbing experience of 'not being there' while at the same time being lifted somewhere other than where we are. Mismatches between the perception of the filmmaker, the camera, and the film-viewer need not, however, be regarded as a problem to be fixed by applying additional degrees of empiricist discipline. In this project I have become interested in the ways in which the encounter with film and the experience of 'not being there' can be applied positively as a phenomenological technique for distancing and displacing ourselves from the ways in which we usually perceive our world (see e.g. Steinbock 2007: 4; Merleau-Ponty 2000; Irving 2013; Schäuble 2016a).

In a widely debated attack on anthropological film, Kirsten Hastrup (1992) argues for the necessity of explicit categories in the production of anthropological knowledge. Treating words and images as ideal types, she claims that while knowledge communicated through film remains iconographic and thin, 'Ethnographic writing, on the other hand, may invoke a degree of reflexivity which enables us to turn knowledge into consciousness, without which we cannot transcend the limitations of established forms, also of difference. With films, differences must be taken at face-value; in writings the context-values that are embodied in the visible differences can be assessed' (Hastrup 1992: 21).

Hastrup provides the example of a series of photographs she took of an exhibition of rams in Iceland. Even though the exhibition was open only to men, she managed to get access to what she soon realised was a competition of sexual potency focused on measuring the size and weight of the ram's testicles. Later, when she developed the photographs – ill-focused, badly lit, lopsided, featuring the backs of men and rams – she was rather disappointed: 'The texture of maleness and sex had been an intense sensory experience, but it was invisible. The reality of the total social event had been transformed into a two-dimensional image, a souvenir' (Hastrup 1992: 9). While Hastrup admits that other photographers might have been able to take better photos, she argues that the 'thick', 'invisible', 'secret' meaning of the event could only be communicated in words (see also Geertz 1993[1973]: 27).

With this book and film, I have turned Hastrup's argument upside-down. Rather than visualising the invisible, I take it to be the responsibility of a filmic ethnography to keep the invisible invisible (see also Suhr and Willerslev 2012; 2013). Instead of taking it to be the business of anthropology to move beyond the divides of cultural difference through the use of abstract categorisation and analysis, I seek to use film as a method for transgressing that which can be contained within categories – to make the differences, wonders, and encounters in the field overflow the categories of my own making.

In this pursuit I am moving away from the idea of film images as offering mirror representations of social life and human subjective seeing. Film, as Vivian Sobchack (1992; see also Castaing-Taylor 1996: 80) points out, is not merely a 'viewed object'. While film is certainly seen and therefore the object of our gaze, it also has a way of seeing which cannot be reduced to the perception of the filmmaker or the spectator. In Sobchack's (1992: 23) words: 'Film cannot be considered a monologic one between a viewing subject and a viewed object. Rather, it is a dialogical and dialectical engagement of [at least] *two* viewing subjects who also exist as visible objects.'

Being exposed to a film image means being exposed to a life over which we often have limited power and which is seldom containable within any given set of categories. For this reason film as a 'viewing subject' equivalent to, yet always and necessarily different from, our own subjective perception, may serve to push us towards a reflection upon our perceptions, categories, and their adequacy in describing the always partly invisible, incongruent, and sometimes even monstrous spectacle we call reality.

Instead of considering film merely as a medium of representation or as an audio-video notebook, we might even think of the camera as a kind of anthropologist in itself. This idea works well with the attempt of pioneering filmmaker and montage theorist Dziga Vertov (1984) to set the camera free to do its work in the production of truthful cinema. Vertov's radical vision was encapsulated by the dictum of the 'kino-eye', simultaneously documenting and constructing reality: a cinema which, as its first move, needed to break away from the mimetic disposition of the camera: 'Until now we have violated the movie camera and forced it to copy the work of our eye. The better the copy, the better the shooting was thought to be. Starting today we are liberating the camera and making it work in the opposite direction – away from copying' (Vertov in Roberts 2000: 19).

Many ethnographic filmmakers have been inspired by the films and writings of Vertov. The cinéma verité movement, developed by Jean Rouch and Edgar Morin (1961), is a direct translation of Vertov's concept of 'Kino Pravda', meaning 'film-truth'. But rather than the intersubjective truth provided by Rouch's living participatory camera (Rouch 2003; see also Rothman 1997: 80), which functions as an extension of the filmmaker's body, Vertov aimed at transcending the intersubjective through montage, thereby obtaining a different vision, extending beyond the subjective viewpoint of the human eye. What was fascinating and useful about the camera for him was not its ability to mimic ordinary human perception or our intersubjective relationships, but rather its capacity to enable us to perceive the world and allow us to be perceived from a point entirely beyond human anchorage. Indeed for Vertov (1984: 15) it was the inability of the camera to see as the human eye – the way in which the camera 'lives and moves in time and space … in a manner wholly different from that of the human eye' – that allowed it to pose questions of social and political relevance.

Might there be a way along these Vertovian lines to think of the camera itself as a kind of film-anthropologist? Certainly I was the one who decided to bring a camera into the field. I decided when to turn it on and off. By now I think of myself as largely in control of the basic operations, how to adjust the focus, correct the white balance, tweak the aperture, and control the audio levels. Most often I prefer to shoot handheld, enjoying the freedom to move the camera towards the objects I am interested in. In the editing I view the material and select certain scenes. I put them together into a filmic structure. But am I fully in charge? When I move around with the camera, is it me who constructs the focal objects, or is it not instead, as James Elkins (1996: 20) puts it, the objects that catch my eye? Most often I seem to select scenes because they surprise me or peak my curiosity. The camera has a life of which I am not fully in control. Often it is the sounds and images it produces that ask me the questions. In this way, categories of thought are moved around and challenged. Since I am unable to fully understand the world presented to me by the camera, we might as well switch roles.

The filmic part of this book is therefore conceived of not only as a video documentation, but as a form of analytical operation in its own right. Its way of viewing provokes insights into the emotional and epistemological dilemmas among patients and healers, but also into the incongruencies between our viewing, the recorded material, and this text. The film is conceived of as the analytical product not only of me the filmmaker, but also of the camera as a mechanical researcher, offering insight while simultaneously posing a number of questions. Some of these questions are expanded in the book, but the elaborations might not always appear sufficient. Sometimes they act as the catalyst for yet further sets of questions.

## *Notes*

1 The differences in opinion between 'Salafis' and 'Sufis' about the possibility of seeing the invisible may be a matter of degree rather than substance. Sometimes critical statements by 'Salafis' or 'Sufis' vis-à-vis each other seem to be intensified by political desires to distance oneself from other believers who are not doing things the correct way. Thus the neo-orthodox Muslims I worked with also recognise that even though the invisible is impossible to see, it is important to approach it through the imagination (*taṣawwur*), for example through remembrance of the punishments of the grave (*dhikr al-mawt*, Al-Ghazali 1989[1058–1111 C.E.]: 37; see also Hirschkind 2006: 183; Pandolfo 2018: 216). Where my interlocutors depart from the perceptual techniques of Sufism is in the degree of how much one may attempt to remember and imagine the invisible. Here my interlocutors advocate a highly cautious approach that constantly emphasises the inability to remember and imagine, and the insufficiency of what is remembered, rather than the intensive cultivation of the imagination reported in Mittermaier's study.

2 See Talal Asad (2003), Phil Zuckerman (2008), Carsten Stage (2011), and Martijn van Beek (2012) for analyses of the complex varieties of secularism.

3 See the Ministry of Social Affairs (2011) and the list of ghettos published by the Ministry of Transport, Building, and Housing (2016) in which income and education were added as criteria. For a discussion of the problematic concept of the 'ghetto' see Wacquant (2008) and Slater (2010).

4 While the overall number of inhabitants in the area has decreased over the last years and the crime rate has decreased, the unemployment rate and the percentage of 'immigrants or descendants of immigrants from non-Western countries' have remained stable (Ministry of Transport, Building, and Housing 2016; Samvirket i Gellerup og Toveshøj 2016).

5 Based on numbers from Statistics Denmark, Hjarn von Zernichow Borberg (2016) points out how, as an example, 77 per cent of second-generation immigrants of Iraqi descent aged 20 to 29 are either employed or in education. Of 'ethnic' Danes in the same age group, 84 per cent are either employed or in education. Despite the traumatic experiences of war and conflict, the illiteracy and unemployment that characterised many first-generation immigrants from Iraq, their children are only 7 per cent behind their Danish peers when it comes to employment and education. 93 per cent of children of immigrants from Iraq perform as well as 'ethnic' Danes at the same age.

6 Lasse Lindekilde (2010) describes how efforts of the Danish state to map environments perceived to be fostering radical Muslim youth in actual fact contribute to religious 'radicalisation' by creating suspicion and mistrust.

7 Literally *majnūn* means 'be-jinned', although this is not often implied in the modern usage of the word. The state of jinn possession is instead described through terms such as *malbūs* (the jinn clothed in the human body), *maskūn* (haunted by the jinn), or *maḍrūb* (paralysed by the jinn). See Maarouf (2007: 139–40) for a description of these terms. See also Badeen and Krawietz (2003) for an analysis of the role of the jinn in the Quran.

8 See also the recently translated work of Tobie Nathan and Isabelle Stengers (2018) that thoroughly problematises the commonly held oppositions between traditional and modern medicine, religion, and science.

# 2

# How to take jinn possession seriously

*Although anthropologists, like painters, lend their bodies to the world, we tend to allow our senses to penetrate the Other's world rather than letting our senses be penetrated by the world of the Other. The result of this tendency is that we represent the Other's world from the outside in a generally turgid discourse which often bears little resemblance to the worlds we are attempting to describe.*

Paul Stoller, 1984

*By 'taking seriously,' I simply mean taking seriously what the people themselves take seriously. This is not usually done in anthropology. Spirits such as those the Yukaghirs claim to exist out there in the world alongside humans and animals and with whom they interact in both waking life and in dreams are generally not accepted by anthropologists as having any reality other than as mental representations, imposed upon the world by indigenous minds as a means of grasping it conceptually and appropriating it symbolically within the terms of a culturally constructed worldview.*

Rane Willerslev, 2007

*I saw with my own eyes a large thing emerging out of the flesh of her back. It was a big gray sphere – a sort of plasm – about six inches across, dark and opaque. I was amazed – delighted. I still laugh with the glee at the realization of having seen it, the Ihamba spirit, and so big! We were all in triumph. The gray thing was actually out in the open ... The patient was now relieved of her sickness ... in ordinary life anywhere, the same thing crops up – among Baptists, rabbis, in the streets of Calcutta, in Lhasa, Tibet, and in the midst of a Sufi prayer meeting. According to the angry old guard of anthropology – which is still here – they're all supposed to be wrong; you should ignore their experience, which never happened anyway ... There are spirits, and we have no business contradicting so many good people around the world.*

Edith Turner, 2006

## Risskov Psychiatric Hospital, February 2011

I am sitting alone in Esther's office. Esther is a nurse at Aarhus University Hospital, Risskov, Centre South, and is part of a specialist team dealing with psychotic illnesses on an outpatient basis. I have been allowed to follow her meetings with Muslim patients.

Aziz and Esther arrive. Aziz is a Lebanese Palestinian, 44 years old, smartly dressed in a black suit, shiny leather shoes, and tie. Esther told me earlier he is suffering from paranoid schizophrenia. Recently he started explaining his illness in terms of affliction by blue magic. This is why she asked if I wanted to see the patient.

'*Al-salāmu ʿalaykum*' – I shake hands with Aziz. Aziz does not shake hands with Esther. Esther told me that this is one of the signs of his religious extremism: 'When Aziz isn't sufficiently medicated he starts doing these things. He doesn't want to shake hands with me because I'm a woman. When he was hospitalised last year he had no problem shaking my hand at all, he even hugged me. He really appreciated it when I visited him. But now we start to see the symptoms again.'

Last year Aziz was committed to the Forensic Psychiatry Section for two months. It happened after a series of violent outbreaks in the mosques of Aarhus. After a short trial Aziz was sentenced to treatment – hospitalised for the sixteenth time since his arrival in Denmark in 1989.

The three of us sit in the small office. Esther sits by the door, with Aziz opposite her on the other side of a small table. She does this routinely so that she can escape if Aziz becomes aggressive. She has never experienced this, but other nurses and social workers have reported problems with him. Esther meets Aziz every Monday to give him his antipsychotic medicine and to check he actually takes the drugs he has been administered. Aziz has to take blood tests every week so that Esther can verify the amount of active psychotropic agents in his body. She estimates that he takes less than a third of the medicine he is supposed to take. Esther fears that Aziz is getting worse and is approaching yet another major psychosis.

'How are you today?' she asks.

'I'm fine. Everything is fine,' Aziz replies.

'Christian is doing a research project and film about healing and Islam. About how Muslims understand healing and illness.'

I explain my project to Aziz. I am interested in understanding how people can be attacked by magic, the evil eye, or become possessed by jinn, and how it is possible to cure these forms of illnesses. Aziz immediately takes over the conversation:

'They give me these pills, they say I have to take pills, but the pills do not help anything. I'm well. I don't have any problems.'

'But *do* you take your pills?' Esther asks.

'Yes, I take them, I always take my medicine, every day,' he replies. 'But the medicine makes me tired.'

'But I can see on the blood tests that you don't take all of it.'

'Yes, I do take it. Because I have to, even though it doesn't work. It's annoying.'

Aziz addresses me.

'I'm not ill. It was magic that made me ill. The medicine only makes me tired. I get so tired. But it doesn't do anything against magic. It was an imam from Vejle [a Danish town], he's very skilled, he removed the magic.

Hurriyet, my ex-wife, she got the magic from her mother in Turkey. Her mother's sister makes these things. *Siḥr.* She earns money from it. Before, I was completely well. I had a good life. Then suddenly, I shifted from being a regular easy-going guy [*stille og rolig*]. But it wasn't me – do you understand? It was something else, someone was inside me, a jinn.'

Aziz tells me the story of how he fell in love with his ex-wife. Aziz was already married when he met her. Aziz's first marriage had been arranged by his older brother, but Aziz and his first wife had problems in their marriage. Some years after the wedding he fell in love with the Turkish woman, Hurriyet. They married secretly (*nikāḥ ʿurfi*) and every day he spent a couple of hours with his second wife. He helped her obtain the highest incapacity benefit possible (*førtidspension*). She was not ill, but he explained what she needed to tell the Danish doctors in order to become eligible for incapacity benefit.

According to Aziz, they had a happy life together for almost ten years. Then two years ago things started to go wrong. Hurriyet became dissatisfied with being the second wife and having to share her husband with another woman. On a visit to her mother in Turkey she received the magic that was later to inflict the jinn possession on Aziz. Years earlier Hurriyet's mother had used the same magic to take control over Hurriyet's father. According to Aziz, Hurriyet wanted a man as her father had been to her mother. She poured the magic into a can of coffee and made Aziz drink it during a picnic at the local cemetery. Like ruins, toilets, and rubbish tips, cemeteries are one of the favourite places for jinn to dwell.

After Aziz drank Hurriyet's coffee at the cemetery, he became obsessed with her. He lost his friends and lost contact with his family. He could think only of Hurriyet and could not stand anyone's company but hers: 'I felt the difference. I could feel that it wasn't me. My [first] wife also felt it. She could sense when it was me and when it was the jinn. I started to speak with different words.'

In the period that followed, several local shaykhs treated Aziz. They read specific healing verses from the Quran (*al-ruqya al-sharʿiyya*) over him, over water he subsequently drank, and over olive oil with which his wife massaged his body in order to purify it. But it did not help. It possibly made things worse by angering the jinn that had taken possession of Aziz. He started to feel hatred towards the shaykhs and the mosque. On one occasion he virtually ransacked a whole mosque in the middle of the Friday prayer:

'I was doing *sujūd* [the position in prayer where the forehead touches the ground]. Then I felt something strange. Something forcing me to bite my hand. I bit hard. I started to scream at the imam. Pig, I cried, you are a pig. He tried to calm me down. I went up to the *minbar* [pulpit] where he was standing.[1] I overturned it and broke it. I dragged him down from the pulpit. I hit him. I tore down the curtains. I ripped out pages from the

Quran. This is not good. I wrecked the whole mosque. It was full. It was the Friday prayer. But they couldn't do anything. I was too strong. The jinn makes me very strong. Four or five policemen came. But then the jinn was clever. It stopped. It wanted me to go with them. They put me in their car. I did nothing. I was sitting in the back. Only when they started to drive it made me give the finger to the crowd standing by the mosque.'

After several violent incidents such as this, culminating in Aziz trying to run over a man in a car park, he was finally put on trial and committed to hospital, where he was subjected to severe antipsychotic medication. During this period both wives visited him independently and brought with them local shaykhs who tried to heal him with Quranic readings. These healing sessions were carried out without the knowledge of the hospital staff, who, according to Aziz, would have prohibited it. The wife would guard the door to the room while the shaykhs attempted to exorcise the jinn.

In the hospital Aziz told his first wife about his secret marriage with his second wife: 'But it was not me who told her, it was the jinn. It wanted to separate me from my wife. She wouldn't believe it. But it told her the address of my other wife and so finally she found out. After this she wanted to divorce me, she left for Canada to stay with her family.'

Even though Aziz's nurse Esther reports that he got better during hospitalisation, Aziz remembers it as one of the saddest periods of his life. He could not go to the mosque and could not maintain his religious practice, and so the jinn could move freely and behave as it liked. For long periods, the staff restrained Aziz in belts. Only when he was finally released could proper treatment begin. The local shaykhs in Aarhus were giving up on him, so he went to a shaykh he knew in a neighbouring town. During the first session the jinn got extremely aggressive and made Aziz throw a desktop computer at the daughter of the shaykh, who could do nothing but call the police to take Aziz away. At the second session, however, the shaykh telephoned a highly esteemed healer in Lebanon who, over the phone, read the Quran for Aziz and entered into conversation with the jinn occupying his body:

'I could feel it evolving. It was heating up. The imam read Surat al-Baqara and al-Zalzala [Quran, chapters 2 and 99]. He asked it if it was a Muslim or an unbeliever. If it was an unbeliever it should move the left finger. If it was Muslim it should move the right. It moved the right. He forced it to go down through the right arm and out to the fingertip. My friend held it there in my finger and pricked my fingertip with a needle so the jinn could get out. I felt relief. I couldn't remember much of what had happened but the Lebanese shaykh told me that the jinn had been talking in Turkish. I don't speak Turkish. It had told him that it was sent by a *sāḥir* [witch or magician] in Turkey. He also told me that the jinn got into me because I drank magic at a cemetery. How could he know this? How could he know that Hurriyet had made me drink that coffee in the cemetery?'

According to Aziz he has been healthy since this event, although life has not been easy on him. Hurriyet does not want to see him anymore. Aziz misses her a lot – they were good for each other until she gave him the magic. Aziz thinks she regrets doing it. She told him she had done something terrible and that now she can't see him anymore. Aziz's first wife has returned from Canada and they live together again. For religious reasons she has decided not to divorce Aziz, but says that he is free to divorce her if he wants. At the moment his main problem is the medicine – it makes him tired and also makes him fat.

'But don't you think that the medicine can also help with the magic?' Esther asks.

'No, it's finished. I don't have problems with magic anymore,' Aziz replies. 'The medicine doesn't work. It's really bothering me – why do I have to take it when I'm well? I know a person who stopped his medicine and after a month he became well. All the imams say the medicine doesn't work.'

Esther defends herself: 'You know I have to administer this system. The court has assessed that you have to take medicine. You have to do it. At least it helps you to sleep.'

## Illness and healing among Muslims in Denmark

What can we do analytically with a story like the one Aziz presented to his nurse and me? Which theories can help us to understand the framework in which he makes sense of his illness? Many contemporary anthropologists argue that we need – in a much more fundamental way than our predecessors – to take seriously the realities of the people we study (Stoller 1984; Turner 2006; Willerslev 2007).

When I began my fieldwork in Aarhus I was deeply inspired by the writings of Amiria Henare, Martin Holbraad, and Sari Wastell (2007: 7–10), who argued for a 'quiet revolution' against the anthropological axiom that people may have different worldviews but ultimately inhabit the same world. What anthropology should be about, they suggested, is turning our own assumptions on their heads so as to make room for imagining the possibility of people inhabiting a multiplicity of worlds. If informants tell us that there is such a thing as a magical 'power powder', the anthropological exercise should not be about translating the idea of a power powder into concepts we already know, but rather, as Holbraad (2007: 204) asserted, about overturning our own assumptions so as to make it possible for us to imagine how powder – in this world – actually *is* power (see also Suhr and Willerslev 2012).

Arguing for a 'multi-ontological' stance, Eduardo Viveiros de Castro (2011: 134) suggested that anthropologists need to allow people to specify the conditions under which what they say is to be understood. According to Viveiros de Castro, this at the outset requires one to set aside one's own world as the framework through which everything else is grasped, and to attempt – at least momentarily – to take at face value the radical alterity presented to us by the other. As Henare, Holbraad, and Wastell (2007: 12) pointed out, this is not an easy task, 'precisely because it turns on the humble … admission that our concepts … must, by definition, be inadequate to translate *different* ones'.

It seems that what these authors were suggesting was indeed a reversal of what many social scientists had been doing for a long time (see also Turner 1993). Viveiros de Castro specifically proposed his dictum of *taking seriously* in opposition to the position of Richard Rorty (1991b: 29), who claimed that: 'We Western liberal intellectuals should accept the fact that we have to start from where we are, and that this means that there are lots of visions which we simply cannot take seriously.' For anthropologists and social scientists studying the spiritual, magical, or religious worlds of others, a primary approach has been to show how beliefs and practices that appear irrational can be analysed and made intelligible by revealing the underlying social mechanisms that are often invisible to the religious practitioners themselves. Often the problem has been phrased along the lines of E. E. Evans-Pritchard's famous study of witchcraft and magic among the Azande in central Africa. Since '[w]itches, as the Azande conceive them, clearly cannot exist', the anthropological problem for Evans-Pritchard (1976[1937]: 18) was how to account for a native reasoning within which otherwise obscure claims about witchcraft could be shown to make sense.

In his later years Evans-Pritchard (1965; 1970) refined his views on magic and religion as he became concerned with mysticism and the transcendental principles shared by Hinduism, Buddhism, and the Abrahamic religions (Barnes 1987; Larsen 2014). Eventually he came to the conclusion that religious experience was best understood by acknowledging the presence of the divine and the validity of religion in a given culture – a position for which he was roundly criticised by colleagues who maintained that a theory about the function of religion needs to be built on concepts far removed from the ways in which religious practitioners themselves would conceive of reality (Luhrmann 2016: 147; Willerslev and Suhr 2018).

The Durkheimian approach offered a framework for understanding religious beliefs and practices as corresponding not to the reality of gods or spirits, but to social reality. For Émile Durkheim (2008[1912]), religion was the very glue that kept society together by securing a moral order. Religion was to be understood as a manifestation and cementing of social solidarity through worship. Sigmund Freud (1989[1933]: 207) held a less optimistic view of religion as a form of illness comparable to childhood neurosis: 'an attempt to master the sensory world in which we are situated by means of the wishful world which we have developed within us as a result of biological and psychological necessities'. In a similar line of thinking, Melford Spiro (1966: 109) argued that religious behaviour serves to reduce unconscious fears and that religion is an institution that functions to reduce anxiety (see also Lehmann and Myers 1993; Malinowski 2004[1948]).

Karl Marx (1975[1844]) launched perhaps the most influential assault on religion by arguing that religious truths are in fact only an expression of and means for the continuation of particular forms of power and social oppression. As he famously declared:

> 'Religion is the sigh of the oppressed creature, the heart of a heartless world, and the soul of soulless conditions. It is the *opium* of the people. The abolition of religion as the illusory happiness of the people is the demand for their real happiness. To call on them to give up their illusions about their condition is to call on them *to give up a condition that requires illusions*. The criticism of religion is, therefore, *in embryo, the criticism of that vale of tears* of which religion is the *halo*' (Marx 1975: 244, emphasis in the original).

In the anthropological study of spirit possession Marxism was taken up by feminists as a tool, not so much to expose the false consciousness of religious or possessed people, but to show how possession can be understood as a strategy of the oppressed to gain agency when no other options are available. In Janice Boddy's (1989: 344–5) work on the *zār* cult in Northern Sudan, she analysed how spirit possession is intimately connected with women's resistance to subordination: 'As the constraints of Islam … gather strength and threaten to undermine women's position, so it may be that women's resistance, or at least their awareness of the threat, is registered in increased acknowledgment of possession' (see also Rothenberg 2004).

In a similar vein, Heba El-Kholy (2002: 183) analysed an epidemic of possession by male American Christian jinn who attacked Egyptian women on the outskirts of Cairo. What was special about American Christian jinn, as compared to Egyptian Muslim jinn, was that while the latter could be exorcised quite easily, American Christian jinn could not be exorcised fully; one could only hope to convert them into Muslim believers. For the women El-Kholy was studying, possession opened up the possibility of refusing to give in to the demands of their husbands. In particular, it seemed that becoming possessed by American Christian jinn was an effective way of avoiding sexual duties in marriage. According to El-Kholy (2002: 186), possession by American Christian jinn established itself as a refuge against male dominance in a social context where women otherwise had little or no right to disobey their husbands, brothers, and fathers.

Theories about possession and religious healing often seem to share a common ambition of somehow exposing underlying invisible structures, real meanings, or logical social mechanisms for why people do what they do and say what they say. The potential violence of such well-meaning attempts to understand and rationalise the perceived 'madness' of others has been analysed by Michel Foucault (1988) in his influential study of the formation of modern psychiatry. As in Plato, we are asked to recognise that behind every appearance lies a hidden truth to be discovered. Realist ethnography of this kind is, as Stoller (1984) points out, precisely about evoking social and cultural unity behind the bits and pieces of data, and hence discovering the invisible truth of reality hidden behind its many appearances. Arguably the search for the 'One in the Many' is still at the heart of much anthropological research. But the work of Henare, Holbraad, Wastell, Viveiros de Castro, and others suggests that the whole enterprise of making sense of other people's worlds in terms of our own concepts is infertile and anthropologically dubious for the way it colonises and risks eliminating the world of the other. As Levinas (1979: 87) points out, attempting to kill alterity is a serious matter, not only because of the danger it inflicts upon others, but because the self too would suffocate and cease to exist through the destruction of the other.

How, then, is it possible to take other people's realities seriously? What does it entail, and what can we learn if we try to take seriously other people's concepts and perceptions of their world? I came to the conclusion that these questions cannot be answered through any amount of logical deductive reasoning. Instead they need to be addressed in the particular, in the midst of the conceptual, perceptual, and emotional interactions taking place in the social field.

## Research seminar, November 2010

I am invited to the psychiatric hospital in Risskov to give a talk about how illness and healing are understood among the Muslims I work with in Aarhus. Present are about forty psychiatrists, psychologists, nurses, and other members of the research staff of the hospital.

After a slow start in 2009, interrupted by administration, travel, and teaching obligations at the university, my fieldwork in Denmark is now well under way. I have decided to do my research at home because of the convenience of living less than ten kilometres away from my interlocutors. Doing fieldwork in Denmark is convenient, but generates special difficulties.

As an anthropologist I have been trained to study the lives of others by participating in people's lives for a prolonged period of time. Active participation enables anthropologists to understand not only how people talk and act, but also how they experience their world. During previous projects in Egypt and Papua New Guinea I had lived and worked with people on an everyday basis. But with this new project in my hometown in Denmark, I have problems connecting. Most of the Muslims I work with live on the other side of a ring road separating the so-called 'ghetto' of Gellerup from the inner city where I live. Scheduling formal interviews and attending sermons or meetings in the mosques is easy, but sharing everyday experiences with my interlocutors beyond that doesn't feel easy at all. To overcome this disjunction, I try to participate as actively as I can in their practices of worship. At least this is how I like to portray my involvement. In actual fact it was my interlocutors who first convinced me to participate. Initially I did everything I could to resist it. 'You say you're an anthropologist,' Abu Samir said, 'then you have to participate. Just try to do the prayer. It's not dangerous, it's like yoga.'

Somehow taking part in prayer seemed much more dangerous than selling camel trips or participating in betel-nut exchanges as I had done in my previous fieldwork. 'If you want to understand Islam, then try it,' Abu Samir said, 'then you'll understand.'

Finally I decided to participate in the prayer, and indeed, as Abu Samir had insistently tried to explain, I suddenly began to understand these worshiping practices in an entirely different way. At the same time, I felt – as Edith Turner (1993: 11) also describes in her experience of 'going native' – that I had somehow really gone over the edge, into some strange and forbidden anthropological territory.

Before the presentation at the psychiatric hospital I do *wuḍū'*, the ritual cleansing used to purify the body before entering prayer. In my car on the way to the seminar I recall what Abu Bilal told me: that I should do two *rak'a* (the prescribed movements in prayer) before the presentation and pray that it will be beneficial and result in *da'wa* (invitation to Islam): 'You must remember that it is the doctors who are ill, they just don't know it. They live in *dunyā* [the earthly visible world] and are so sure about it. They cannot believe that there is something else. It's *jāhiliyya* [ignorance of God's guidance].'

I am divided. For some reason I can't get myself to do the two *rak'a*, but I pray in my own way that somehow the presentation will be beneficial. I have rehearsed the presentation several times with Abu Bilal and others from the mosque, and have tried to organise the talk in a similar format to that used by Abu Bilal in his lectures. My attempt is to incorporate and implicate the psychiatrists and nurses in an act of participant observation and then to observe the kinds of questions, answers, resonances, and dissonances that might arise from bringing neo-orthodox Islamic theology into contact with Danish psychiatry. As such it is a miniature experiment in the practice of 'taking seriously' – an attempt not to filter, translate, or in other ways reduce the perspectives and understandings of my Muslim collaborators.

'When we are going to start a talk like this, then it's a good idea to start by saying a little prayer, a *du'ā'*.'

I recite and explain the *du'ā'* used before any major activity.

'First we pray for God to protect us against the evil demons which could attack us while we are sitting here. Then we pray that whatever will be said in this room will be said in the name of God. Lastly we send our prayers to the prophets of God.'

At least as a rhetorical device for opening my presentation, the small supplication has worked. The psychiatrists, psychologists, and nurses seem attentive.

'It's important to say this prayer because now we are going to talk about the evil demons and what they do. The greatest trick of Iblis – the greatest, first, and worst of the demons – is the way he persuades people into believing that he doesn't exist. The devil, Iblis, or *shayṭān*, as he is also called, was originally a jinn – a spirit – who refused to obey the will of God. While humans are made of clay, he was created from fire, and for this reason he thought himself better than humans and didn't want to welcome humans into the world. Due to this arrogance – *kibr*, which is one of the worst sins in Islam – Iblis is irrevocably condemned to hell. But Iblis has *ḥasad*, envy: he cannot accept that humans will go to paradise, and for this reason he tries as hard as he can to drag humans with him to hell. The method is chiefly by creating doubt about the truth, by convincing people that there are other gods than God, or by convincing people that they themselves are in fact gods. Worship of anyone else than God is *shirk*, and *shirk* is a certain ticket to hell.'

'Now, God is almighty. God has created everything and holds the power to change everything. So why does God allow Iblis to fool the humans? It is because humans are placed in this world – *dunyā* – as a test. The test is simple. Are we able to take up the task we have been given? The task is to worship God. Worship is many things. It is, for example, the small supplication we did before starting this presentation. It is the five daily prayers, it is *ḥajj* (the pilgrimage), it is *zakāt* (alms giving), and the fasting during Ramadan (*ṣawm*). But it is also all the small things we do in daily life. If we try to do them the right way, namely the way assigned to us by God through the holy scriptures and the example of the Prophet, then they become acts of worship. That we sleep in a certain way, that we make a certain supplication before entering sleep and when we wake up, when we eat, when we start our car, that we have sex in a certain way and in the name of God, that we enter the toilet with the left foot first and exit with the right. We need to do all this for the sake of God. It is not, however, because God needs it. It is because we need it. Through submitting ourselves to God, we are rewarded with paradise in this life and in the afterlife.'

'In short, worship is about including the hidden, invisible, and unseen – *al-ghayb* – in all the actions we take in this visible world. But what does this mean, to believe or have faith in the invisible?'

'It means believing that there is a life after death – *al-ākhira* – and that we will inevitably end up either in hell or in paradise. Part of hell lies in the sun and part of it lies deep below the surface of the earth, but it is impossible for us to see it. Paradise lies up beyond the first sky and continues upwards until the seventh sky, but we cannot see it.'

'It also means believing that there are angels: creatures made of light, creatures who unlike humans submit themselves entirely to the worship of God. And it means believing that there are jinn: creatures made of fire who live in a parallel world to the world of humans. They are born and have children. Many of these jinn are good, practising Muslims. But some of them have become evil, *shayāṭīn*, and together with Iblis they have devoted themselves to the task of dragging the believers away from the truth.'

'Most importantly, it means to be absolutely certain that there is only one God – *lā ʾilāha ʾillā l-Lāh*. God is *ghayb* – impossible to reach through the senses – for the good reason that we would be crushed if we could see him. So great is the beauty and glory of God. In fact we would be crushed if we could see just a tiny bit of paradise. If, for example, just the veil of one of the beautiful women of paradise were to show in this world, then all the space between the earth and up to the first sky would explode in divine light.'

At this point in the presentation I begin to feel as though I am losing members of the audience. An Iranian psychiatrist interrupts the talk. He asks me where I got this information from. He is not himself a practising Muslim, but nevertheless he was brought up in Islam. He has never heard anything like the things I am recounting here. 'Surely it must be a very small minority of Muslims who hold these beliefs?' he asks. I point out that what I say here is based on my fieldwork among neo-orthodox Arab, Turkish, Iraqi, Afghan, and Somali Muslims in Aarhus. What I present is by no means representative of all Muslims. The Iranian psychiatrist suggests that he could put me in contact with some Muslim theologians with a deeper and more nuanced knowledge of what Islam is about. He fears that if I continue to focus on the superstitious beliefs held by these Muslims, it will become very difficult to generalise on the basis of my findings.

I thank him – it would probably be highly useful for me to meet these Muslim theologians. But I also respond by arguing that the value of anthropological knowledge is not necessarily determined by its scale of applicability. Rather what anthropologists often seek is to obtain specific knowledge from long-term collaboration with relatively few individuals, which in turn may be used to challenge and move around with social theories on a larger scale.

Is this taking the 'ontology' of the other seriously? To reduce in this way the universal truth of my collaborators to just one particular truth – the truth as it appears to them? Perhaps I am stumbling into some of the difficulties in the radical constructivist position of Henare, Holbraad, and Wastell (2007). How do we take the ontology of our field-collaborators seriously if they insist that their truth is the only truth available? And how do we present such a truth to audiences who, likewise, seem to be equally sure of the universal validity of their own conceptions of reality? What lies on the reverse side of the radical constructivist position, which holds that people do not in fact live in the same world but in radically different worlds?

As Henare, Holbraad, and Wastell (2007: 14–15) asserted, to conceive of a different world 'is to *conceive* it – to think it into being, because thought here just is being. Conception is a mode of disclosure … that creates its own objects, just because it is one and the same with them, so to "see" these objects is to create them' (emphasis in the original). Constructivism, as presented by Henare, Holbraad, and Wastell, appears to be a particular radical form of relativism. But how then is relativism different from universalism – are they just two sides of the same coin? Does this *truth of truths* not necessarily deny the possibility of an alternative universal truth such as that presented by my Muslim interlocutors?

The attempt to break out of the 'truth behind the many' (Stoller 1984: 104) seems to have gone full circle. Doubt is sneaking into my presentation. I am flipping between either incompatible or completely meaningless positions. Am I hypocritical? Have I pretended to deliver the universal truth of Islam to these psychiatrists when in reality I know how partial and situated this view of Islam is? Or am I hypocritical to distance myself from the ontology of my field-collaborators – was this not the only way to get an understanding of their particular universalism? I am not settled in my opinions on this. Perhaps the real problem is that to some extent I have started to believe in the things my interlocutors tell me. Not to believe while participating in prayer seemed almost impossible. Was I voluntarily letting myself be brainwashed, or had my heart finally been opened to receive the invisible truth? After the intervention of the Iranian doctor I try to continue a little differently:

'I imagine some of you may be thinking that this anthropologist must be crazy. But I think that if you – as a researcher, anthropologist, nurse, or psychiatrist – really want to understand how very believing and practising Muslims experience the world, then you must somehow try to put yourself into it. The greatest trick of the devil is to convince us that he doesn't exist.

Denial of the existence of the invisible, of God, angels, jinn, and the afterlife is the work of the devil. So if you doubt what I am telling you now, then you should try to imagine that this doubt doesn't stem from yourself. At least this is how many of your Muslim patients would understand the situation. Doubt is inserted into you by small invisible devils that flow through your blood and fill the airspace around you, whispering the doubt into your consciousness – *waswās al-shayāṭīn*. They do this because doubt (*shakk*) about the existence of God and the unseen leads directly to hell. Perhaps you cannot hear their whispering, but if you pray and ask God for protection then it is possible that with time you will be able to separate your own consciousness and will from the whisperings of *shayāṭīn*.'

'*A'ūdhu bi-l-Lāh* – God protect us. When we say this supplication, submit ourselves, and pray to God for his help, you should imagine how the airspace surrounding you is instantly purified – how all the evil spirits who were flocking around you, competing to whisper the most horrible and dangerous lies, with tremendous force are pushed away from your body. Instead angels descend from above and sit around us and upon us and upon each other and bring our prayer all the way up through the seven skies to God. And God, *in shā' Allāh* (God willing), rewards us for this. Every time we mention the name of God, pray, or do a good deed for the sake of God, then a reward ten times as great as our deed is sent down to us. This opens our hearts so that we become capable of receiving the truth about the invisible world.'

## Esther's office, March 2011

Aziz has left the office. This was the third of Esther's meetings with Aziz that I have attended, and this is the third time I have heard his story about the jinn, the magic, and how he was healed by the words of the Quran. I have started to film the sessions. Aziz was happy to accept being filmed. I think he agreed to participate in the film in order to show the doctors and the people in the mosques the real reason he became so violent. During our film recordings it seems clear Aziz is trying to use me as a kind of truth-witness to the reality of jinn and magic. Filming in this way becomes another modality of participant observation – an enquiry into social life that does not only passively observe, but actively participates as a special and complicit form of witnessing (Marcus 1998). After Aziz has left the office and the camera has been turned off I ask Esther what she thinks of the story of how Aziz taught his ex-wife to say the right things in order to obtain incapacity benefits from the state.

'I think it is very common,' she answers. 'A while ago Aziz told me about a psychiatrist in Copenhagen they pay to help them say the right things to doctors in order to become eligible for incapacity benefits. Aziz mentioned the name and address. I checked and there is a psychiatrist with that name. I think it does happen. Unfortunately.'

I ask if she has patients where this could be the case. Even though she is convinced that it happens, she doesn't believe that any of her patients would be faking in this way: 'Look at Aziz, he's clearly insane.'

I nod, I think I agree: 'But it seems that he's saying all this to get rid of the medicine, right, to prove to you that he isn't ill anymore?'

'That's true,' Esther replies, 'but if that meant he would have to go out to work, then he might be presenting his story differently.'

We are both puzzled by the consistency of Aziz's story. In Esther's vocabulary this is a case of highly developed and coherent psychotic delusions. Esther knows the antipsychotic drugs help reduce the delusions. When he is sufficiently medicated and not exposed to the shaykhs in the mosque, he is able to see through the delusions and recognise them for what they are.

Here Esther appears to firmly believe in the efficacy of biomedicine and its adequacy as an explanatory framework for understanding the suffering of her patient. She acknowledges that the occult beliefs of patients may have, for them, what she calls a 'reality character'. In the treatment she attempts to not directly oppose or contradict the beliefs of her patients, as to do so would make it very difficult to ensure compliance. Instead she attempts to build an alliance between the self-diagnosis of patients and the psychiatric diagnosis. Sometimes she directly encourages people to seek religious guidance or relief in prayer, if this is what the patients themselves appear to believe in. The psychotherapeutic drugs are then presented as a means of supporting the patients in this endeavour by reducing anxiety, emotional stress, nightmares, etc.

As in the work of several other nurses I follow at the hospital, the strategy of building an alliance between the life-world of the patient and reality as understood in the psychiatric framework only partially succeeds. Due to the limited time available for meetings with patients, it is often impossible to reach an in-depth understanding of what the patients themselves believe they are suffering from. But perhaps too much of such knowledge would make it difficult for the nurses to intervene, making the patient an expert in her or his own suffering with less need for external intervention. The most effective strategy is rather for the nurses to obtain only some knowledge of the world of the patient, which can then be made intelligible within the vocabulary of psychiatric healthcare. Consider a short interchange between another nurse and an Afghan woman diagnosed with 'schizoaffective psychosis (depressive type), PTSD, and chronic headache':

Nurse: 'How about the psychotic thoughts?'

Patient: 'They are still here. This Friday in the kitchen. Three or four persons, I could not hear what they were saying. They were just mumbling.'

Nurse: 'For how long?'

Patient: 'Maybe four minutes. I couldn't recognise them. I was frightened. My heart starts to throb. I shake. I call my husband. I know it's not real, but I believe it's real.'

Nurse: 'This is a sign of health. You know how to place the experience. That the experience has the character of being real.'

For the nurse, the ability of the patient to affirm the 'unreality' of her experience testifies to her compliance with the treatment. After the discussion the nurse decides to increase the medication, which seems to have a positive effect. The patient is very hesitant about this decision, but accepts it. She is in a vulnerable position since she needs to stay on sickness benefits in order to have sufficient time to learn Danish, so that she can pass the 'national attachment' tests required for obtaining citizenship in Denmark. Without a Danish passport she cannot travel to Canada where most of her family lives. After meeting with the patient, the nurse tells me she actually thinks loneliness is the biggest problem this patient is suffering from. Loneliness, however, is not something that Danish psychiatric healthcare is able to do much about.

Another nurse tells me something similar:

'I can't just tell the patient that I don't understand the medicine and that I wouldn't dare to take it myself. Shouldn't we just go to the cinema once a week instead? But I think the relationship is crucial. People have lost their trust in the world. For them, what is important is to experience that it is possible to trust and attach to other people. But because we don't have time, there's a tendency to focus exclusively on medication. We have our key tasks: to diagnose and to find the correct medication. Medication, this is the guys who get the money, this is where you have evidence. Nobody receives money for the soft things, here there's no evidence, it's just stuffing. But for me to establish a relationship of trust is the most important. If the patient doesn't trust me, then I cannot help her.'

It continues to puzzle me how the nurses seem to combine such belief and non-belief in biomedicine. In front of the patients there is not a shred of doubt in their statements about the positive effects of the medicine. But after their meetings with patients are over, they often tell me about the problems of not being able to control the side effects of the drugs, that the drugs seem to be working in unpredictable ways on different ethnic groups, the difficulties in poly-pharmacy, and the specific problems related to the generic drugs, which are the only ones most of their patients can afford. While Aziz's nurse Esther, in most contexts, appears to be a firm believer in the efficacy of psychiatric drugs, she is also a devoted and practising Buddhist. When she gets stressed herself, she takes a meditation retreat in a Nepalese monastery and takes Tibetan herbal medicines. After a meeting with a patient, she tells me that with some of her patients she sometimes thinks that if demons exist, then these patients must be possessed by them.

Even though the Afghan woman with 'schizoaffective psychosis (depressive type), PTSD, and chronic headache' clearly acknowledges the unreality of her psychotic experiences in her meetings with her nurse, it is quite obvious she spends time every day protecting herself and her children from the evil attacks of jinn and magic. When I ask her, it seems she is also struggling to find out whether what she sees and hears are in fact jinn or ghosts who have travelled with her all the way from Afghanistan. 'It's just our culture,' she explains, 'I know it's not real.'

## Abu Samir packs his furniture, February 2011

Abu Samir is a refugee from civil war in the Middle East. He married a Danish woman who converted to Islam as a teenager. Together they have two children. Abu Samir and his wife are very pessimistic about the future for Muslims in Denmark, and despite the upheavals, the civil war, and the lack of social security they have decided to move back to the country he left. For them to keep the children in Denmark is simply too dangerous. Just before his departure in early February 2011, Abu Samir tells me about the illness among the Muslim population that is contracted from living in the Danish welfare state.

'Lots of people in this country – too many people, the refugee people – they try to become pensioners, to receive incapacity benefits. But most of them are lying. They try to show that they have a psychological problem and step by step they start to believe that they are sick. But they are not. He makes this problem for himself when he goes to the hospital and they start to give him medicine and he starts to take this medicine. Normally he's capable of using his brain, but when he starts to use the medicine, he loses control: control over his body, his brain, his life. He gets the benefits, but he loses himself. This is the problem here. Most of them go to the RCT [Rehabilitation Centre for Torture Victims] and ask them to look at their psychological problems. Eighty-five per cent of them don't have anything. He tries to show the people that he is seriously sick, and in the hospital they listen to him and start to give him medicine. That medicine, if he doesn't take it, he will be in trouble. Most of them take the medicine and it takes them from being normal to not normal. I hope those who try to get the pension start to be clearer to themselves, because this is not allowed in Islam. To lie and to take money for lying. It is a catastrophe. You sell yourself and your life for nothing.'

I ask Abu Samir about the time he also visited the doctor.

'Before, I also had some psychological problems. I was stressed. The doctor gave me medicine. The medicine took me out of control. I went to him and fought him. I said to him: "I am sick, I don't want this kind of sickness as well, I don't want to become sicker, to become a drug addict." If you use these things you lose. They don't know that they lose, but step by step the drugs start to control their lives.'

'But can't the medicine sometimes be helpful?' I ask.

'The problem is that the Danish system drags people down. They want us to be like them, but we cannot.'

## Amir, April 2011

I use my weight to keep Feisal's hand down. More than twenty-six jinn have been hiding in his body, and now Amir has gone into Feisal again. Amir tries to protect himself against the verses of the Quran by making the sign of the cross with his hand. I force the hand down to the floor, but he is strong. When Feisal still lived in Bosnia he was a karate master. Feisal became ill after moving to Denmark and getting married two years ago. Somehow his possession appears to be connected to his living in this country. Abu Bilal reads louder. Feisal's feet shake violently, his fingers stretch out in shifting gestures and signs, and his head rolls from side to side, eyes wildly staring up towards the ceiling. The muscles in the belly and the legs contract in odd ways. The whole thing has been going on for around half an hour.

It feels strange to be physically preventing a jinn from protecting itself with the sign of the cross. Is this participant observation? Is this allowed? Feisal has asked me to help in his struggle against the jinn, but am I entitled to forcibly prevent a jinn spirit from practising a certain religion? If I try to take the reality of my human interlocutors seriously, should I then not also take the reality of the spirits seriously? Does the invisible face of the jinn not place exactly the same ethical demand on me as its human host? Staring into the unsteady eyes of Amir possessing Feisal, I have no time to think about these questions. I press his hand to the ground, Abu Bilal raises his voice, the body shudders with pain.

When Abu Bilal first started to read, a Bosnian jinn appeared, but when it finally gave up and left the body, it was immediately replaced by Amir. Amir speaks Arabic in a deep guttural voice. This has happened at previous exorcisms as well, but it continues to shock me, because Feisal does not speak Arabic. The secular rational analyst in me immediately starts to produce possible explanations: this is something Feisal has learned; he has watched it on YouTube and now performs it for us; he is unconsciously faking this possession to attract attention to his suffering; or, as I once heard, certain states of consciousness may in fact open up to passive languages hidden deep within our brains. At the same time I recite a supplication for protection, just in case the jinn might come out and attack us. This is the greatest risk in exorcisms. In Egypt several cases have been reported where a jinn was exorcised by a shaykh but then took the shaykh into possession and made him beat the patient to death (Drieskens 2008: 195).

Amir shuffles the verses of the Quran and insistently claims that prophet Solomon was in fact an unbeliever. On previous occasions Amir told us that he himself is an Arab Christian.

'Take the *shahāda* [the Islamic creed]' cries Abu Bilal, trying again to force the jinn to convert to Islam. This is the easiest and most common way to exorcise a jinn. A truly believing Muslim jinn has to recognise that it may not interfere in the world of the humans. A converted jinn will happily leave the human body, even though it often means it will face death when returning to its own world, where its kin will seek to avenge its treachery.

'No one has the right to force another to become a believer,' cries Amir citing yet another verse from the Quran.

'Then I shall burn you out of this body.' Abu Bilal begins reciting again. The body seems to be writhing in pain.

'Say: there is no other god but God, *lā ʾilāha ʾillā l-Lāh*.'

The jinn finally starts to take the creed, but then refuses to say the last part.

'Say: Muhammad is the Prophet of God,' cries Abu Bilal.

Amir starts to weep. He cannot hold up against the pressure anymore. Then suddenly he seems to disappear, and Feisal returns.

## My car, February 2011

Abu Bilal and I are driving back from the mosque. The first rays of sun are lighting the sky. It is seven in the morning. Together with twelve others from the mosque, we have spent the last two hours of the night performing the voluntary night prayer, *qiyām al-layl*, followed by the first obligatory prayer that takes place before daybreak, *ṣalāt al-fajr*. The people from the mosque try to do this at least once every week. Abu Bilal says that ideally, he should do it every night as the Prophet did, but one voluntary night prayer a week is the least we can do in praise of God.

I ask Abu Bilal about the incident in which Aziz became possessed by the jinn and wrecked the mosque last year.

'He had a very strong jinn,' says Abu Bilal, 'but the problem now is that he takes all this medicine. He became addicted to it – like a junkie. You can see him when he walks – it is as if he's sleeping. We had many problems with him. He didn't just smash up the mosque. At *ṣalāt al-fajr* he tried to run people over on the road. He's very dangerous. We tried to read for him – me, Hosna, and Muhammad. We helped his wife. And when he was hospitalised we visited him and brought him sandwiches. Now we have told him he cannot come to the mosque anymore.'

I have stopped the car in front of Abu Bilal's apartment. He stares out through the window. It seems to be hurting him to talk of these events. I tell him Aziz now thinks he is well again, but that he's very unhappy about having to take the medicine. He wants me to tell the doctors that he doesn't need to take it anymore.

'No,' Abu Bilal interrupts me, 'it's good that he takes the medicine. Don't help him to stop the medicine. It's not only a jinn that caused the problems. There's also something else. From the very beginning something wasn't normal. I think he has a multiple personality disorder. When he sat with us he could be nice and happy and suddenly he would become angry and call us horrible things. Sometimes I think he knows what he's doing. I'm not sure. If you're going to write about this then you have to understand that no matter how much you do, you'll never find out what is wrong with him.'

Abu Bilal gets out of the car. Questions are growing in my mind as I drive back through the awakening city. The shaykh who usually tells me about the danger of taking psychiatric drugs and warns about how Danish psychiatric healthcare is making people sick, claiming that true Muslim believers simply cannot get mentally ill, is now asking me to make sure Aziz keeps taking his drugs. He even offers an additional psychiatric diagnosis. Abu Bilal is clearly scared about what might happen if Aziz is not sufficiently drugged.

## Not taking things too seriously

What do anthropologists mean by taking other people's ontology seriously? In their meetings with patients, both Muslim shaykhs and Danish nurses seem to take their treatment and the world of knowledge it is based on extremely seriously. When talking to their patients or to me about their treatment in general terms, there is no doubt about the efficacy of their healing. Yet when asked about particular cases, doubt and uncertainty seem to be the rule rather than the exception. When I present my research project to nurses at the hospital, many of them tell me I have simply come to the wrong place: 'Healing, no. There is no healing here.' Perhaps *taking seriously*, then, means *not taking things too seriously* (see Luhrmann 2000: 26; Willerslev 2013a). At least it must involve taking ambiguity seriously as something that characterises the often-paradoxical statements of healers and patients. Venturing into these territories, no certainty seems to be granted, whether for the patients, nurses, or the shaykhs. For healing to occur it seems necessary, however, that the healers take on the role of seers and knowers who are able to see through the problems reported by the patient, to identify their invisible causes, and then relate these causes to an external body of knowledge and healing power. Often the healers appear to establish their authority by exposing the initial self-diagnosis of the patient as being in some way insufficient.

When Feisal, who was possessed by at least twenty-six jinn, first approached Abu Bilal and me, he showed us how they were constantly moving around in his leg muscle. Whenever the name of God was pronounced above the muscle, it would start moving and contracting. Later the same started to happen in his wife's leg muscle. After the first healing session Abu Bilal could confirm that Feisal was definitely possessed by several very strong jinn of diverse nationalities and religions. Furthermore, he could confirm that Feisal had also been a victim of evil magic, probably placed on him by a witch in Bosnia. But according to Abu Bilal, neither jinn nor magic caused the contractions in the muscle. This was more likely a physical reaction caused by the psychological problems that sometimes accompany severe cases of possession: 'Don't think about it too much, Feisal, try not to think about it.'

Neither the framework of Islam for understanding illness and healing in terms of magical and divine agencies, nor that of modern Western psychiatric healthcare seems to conform to what Evans-Pritchard (1976) would describe as a closed system of belief where each and every occurrence is subsumed within an overall logic. In some ways everything seems capable of being explained in terms of the psychiatric and Islamic frameworks; but practitioners in both systems of thought often seem occupied with questioning possible explanations.

I am not sure how to make sense of this. What philosophers such as Merleau-Ponty and Levinas would call the invisible or the unknown definitely seems to be at stake here. Foucault's (1988: 262ff) analysis of the way in which madness is rendered visible and objectified as afflictions to be cured provides another framework for understanding the interactions between healers and their patients. Diagnoses such as jinn possession, psychosis, and schizophrenia can be understood as attempts at objectification. But at the same time, both the Muslim healers and the health professionals in the psychiatric system seem acutely aware of how the destructive and healing powers they are dealing with exceed the categories they have available. What exactly is the relation between the visible and invisible, the known and the unknown in these healing encounters?

Seen through Durkheimian optics, possession could be understood as a specific form of magic in which individuals are able to assert their will against the social norms of their community. Exorcism, in such a model, then becomes a way of society reinstating the moral order in the individual.

The body of the possessed individual becomes a kind of reverse idol – the personification of evil – through the destruction of which society worships and reproduces itself. Yet the many instances in which Muslim healers, possessed patients, and ordinary believers actively sow their own doubts about the reality of particular cases of possession do not seem to fit into a Durkheimian logic (see also Bubandt 2014). Rather, they seem to be actively destroying the possibility for idolatry.

Another way to understand the Islamic treatment of jinn possession could be to apply theological tools such as Jean-Luc Marion's (2002: 150) concept of distance: the idea that distance is a necessary requirement for worship (see also Horner 2005: 54). Using the analytical terms of Marion, we might conceive of the body of the possessed not as an idol, but as a kind of icon; a peculiar kind of visual display pointing towards something outside the realm of the visible. The uncertainty created around the body seems to enforce an opening into the invisible and unknown. Levinas (1985) has argued that the invisibility of the other and of God is necessary for devotion and love to occur. The uncertainty and doubt created around the possessed body – its invisibility – might be exactly what makes it possible to use possession to facilitate devotion and submission to God.

If such an analysis could account for the engagement with the jinn among the Muslims I work with, how then can I understand the psychiatric treatments? Are they also involved in such a complicated relationship with the invisible? Can a similar dynamic between doubt, faith, and invisibility be identified in Esther's attempts to make Aziz believe in and accept the psychotropic medication he is sentenced to take?

Viveiros de Castro, Henare, Holbraad, and Wastell also talk about 'not taking too seriously', but not at all in this sense, that somehow doubt or a degree of scepticism could be the vehicle or facilitator of belief in a supreme invisible agency (see also Willerslev and Pedersen 2010). As Viveiros de Castro (2011: 133) writes: 'While we strive to take seriously things that are far from or outside of us, almost all of the things that we must not take seriously are near to or inside of us.' For Viveiros de Castro, one of the things that is near to us and that we should therefore not take seriously is the very idea of 'belief'. Belief is part of the world of the 'Nazis' and the 'Western liberal intellectuals' who subscribe to what he calls 'suprasensible absolutism' (Viveiros de Castro 2011: 133, 143–4), a dogma which, not unlike Evans-Pritchard's notion of a closed system of belief, holds that 'even if it is false, it is true'. By contrast, what we need to take seriously, according to Viveiros de Castro, is the alternative world of all the others, the so-called 'people on the far bank of the river', especially the Amazonians, who in a 'multiperspectival' world find truth only in magical efficacy. As Holbraad (2012) also asserts, for these people life is not a matter of achieving or deconstructing belief in a certain representation of the world, but about the effects of truths and how multiple worlds are objectively produced through the creation of truth.

Asad (2003: 23, 55) launched a similar attack on religious studies obsessed with notions like faith and belief, notions that in his view should be understood as 'secular' techniques, which achieved their importance in the modern attempt to separate the spiritual from the realm of reason. Also Stanley Tambiah (1990: 4ff) notes how religion was originally 'something one felt and did', rather than an option one could choose to believe in. Both Tambiah and Asad link the 'birth of belief' as a matter of growing importance to the Protestant Reformation and the European period of Enlightenment, after which religion as an institution gradually became objectified as a system of ideas with particular histories that could be the object of scientific scrutiny.

While Asad builds his critique of belief within the framework of Foucault, for his part Viveiros de Castro finds support in Gilles Deleuze. With the theoretical tools of Deleuze, Viveiros de Castro proposes a notion of seriousness not as respecting people's beliefs but as 'refraining from actualizing the possible expressions of alien thought and deciding to sustain them as possibilities' (Candea 2011: 147). Viveiros de Castro still does not find 'belief' to be worthy of being taken seriously, however. What then do we do if 'belief', 'faith', and even 'existential doubt' are what our interlocutors take seriously, or at least say they take seriously? This debate seems to have become rather convoluted. The more I try to take my interlocutors seriously, the more sceptical I become of the whole anthropological discourse of taking seriously.[2]

'Witches, as at least a radical constructivist philosophy would conceive them, could in fact exist.' Is this what the school of *taking seriously* has taught anthropology? Or is this just another, possibly more advanced way of dispelling the exotic phenomena of the worlds of others? Edith Turner (1992: 148–9) takes a different stance here. During fieldwork in Zambia she saw a real spirit emerge from a patient's back. To her, the question is not about the objective existence of these spirits. If we cannot see them it is simply because we do not dare to see them, a kind of positivist denial fuelled by our academic anxieties about going native (Turner 1993: 9; see also Mittermaier 2011: 89).

For Turner, taking seriously must involve at least a degree of going native, living a piece of life together, and letting perceptions overflow. Taking seriously is not possible when perceiving the other entirely from a distance. At least some amount of proximity, participation, and sharing is required. Allowing the invisible and the other to intrude into the analysis is 'serious' anthropology.

I have tried to take seriously in precisely this way, but still I have been unable to actually see a spirit. Invisible spiritual substance appears to abound in some of my film recordings of Islamic exorcisms, yet all I can see are the visible facades. Below the facades things are happening, but the footage does not allow me to grasp precisely what they are.

A few times I did have some strange experiences, but not of such a definitive kind that I could say afterwards that this was in actual fact a spirit. One evening, just before falling asleep after a particularly intense day of filming, a soft white sphere, approximately the size of my body, appeared to descend from above. It slowly covered and partly entered my body. I had my eyes closed and kept them closed in order not to lose the vision. At that point, certain sentences emerged that at the time appeared to be important messages about things that happened when I was a child. It was a strange, yet also joyful and somehow weightless experience that kept me awake for most of the night. The next morning I was not able to tell whether it had been a dream or something I had actually seen. Months later I discussed the experience with Abu Samir. He could not give any definitive answers: it could have happened simply because I was exhausted, it could have been a normal dream sent from the *nafs*, and it could also have been a form of vision (*ru'yā*). He did not think it was the work of the jinn, since they usually come from the sides or below when they enter people's dreams. Whatever it was, he urged me not to think too much about it.

Some of my interlocutors also told of strange visual experiences, and a few told me their experiences of seeing the jinn. One man had seen a jinn praying on the carpet in the mosque, and a social worker of Palestinian background once saw a group of ugly old female jinn during a visit to the home of one of her patients. Yet both of them also told me about the doubts they had of their visions. In addition, the social worker explained how she tried to forget the disturbing faces of the jinn, since the remembrance of them often interrupted her thoughts and made it difficult for her to do her work. Is there a way in which the anthropological method of taking seriously might involve such partial visions, fluctuating degrees of belief, and even existential doubt? Is there a way in which taking seriously might lead to recognition of the invisible as something beyond our perceptual grasp, the recognition of the spiritual world as an enigmatic paradox that forces our capacity for seeing and knowing outside of itself?

'What we can grasp is our own assumptions,' Henare, Holbraad, and Wastell (2007: 15–16) assert. 'This, we would argue, is an enabling (perhaps the only enabling) starting point for conceptual creation. How far can we go and in what direction must we change our own concepts before we too can assent to our informants' initially bizarre claims?'

## My house, afternoon, March 2011

I stand alone in the rain and light a cigarette. Real spirits exist. Psi exists. 'Spirit-energy is everywhere.' I just read Turner's (2006) article 'Advances in the Study of Spirit Experience'. The rain drips down my face and hand. My cigarette gets wet but the fire dries the moisture from the inside, releasing it as a mist.

'Every raindrop is carried down by an angel,' says Muhammad, my Somali friend who studies engineering. I look around me. Angels are everywhere. Thousands of them. Pouring down from an imperceptible starting point up in the grey sky, bent north slightly by gusts of wind. The wind, also carried by angels. Thousands and thousands of drops explode in small bursts as they hit the asphalt, the leaves, and the roof of the carport; sliding over the plastic, pouring from the edges in streams, and splashing onto the hard surface where puddles are combined into streams flowing towards the drain. I feel the warm smoke filling my lungs. Inhaling, exhaling.

'This is the whispering of *shayāṭīn*,' Abu Bilal says. 'They want you to do it. To do haram – what is forbidden by God.'

'With time you will learn to distinguish their whispering from your own thoughts,' says Abu Seinan.

'This body is *amāna*, it has been entrusted to you by God, so you should take care of it. When you smoke the angels flee, they don't like the scent of it. And then *shayāṭīn* can move as freely as they like.'

I remember putting the boys to sleep yesterday evening. Three days ago, my youngest son started having nightmares. A dark figure tried to drag him somewhere. He was terrified. He no longer wants to sleep in his bed. I tell him his brother is here too – he is already asleep – and I am here to take care of him. Nothing here can harm him; there is nothing to be afraid of.

His eyes are wide open, staring out into the dark room. The pictures of the elephant, the spider, and the stingray that we took on our holiday last year are hanging in their frames above him. In the darkness their colours and contours are indistinguishable; they take on weird forms.

'The angels cannot enter a room where pictures of humans or animals are displayed,' says Abu Bilal. 'Then *shayāṭīn* can do what they want.'

I remember how he purified the bedroom of the Bosnian girl. The posters of *Sex and the City* and Marilyn Monroe, and the photographs of her and her sister had to be removed. She was lucky she was not already possessed by a jinn. In my son's bedroom pictures of animals and humans hang everywhere.

What is it my five-year-old boy sees in the dark? It is way past the time he should be asleep, but he cannot sleep. 'This room has nightmares,' he cries, 'I don't want to sleep here. It's not good.' Am I right to ridicule his fear by trying to convince him that there really is nothing here that can harm him? I try to comfort him, holding him in my arms.

Abdel Rahman told me that this was a real danger. If you deal with the jinn they will try to harm you. Perhaps not you personally, but perhaps they will start with your family. And they are patient. They do not attack immediately. Perhaps they sneak into your car on your way home, first observing your life before they start making plans. This is how it happens.

When we had the discussion, I felt divided. Something inside me said okay, Abdel Rahman says this, but I don't really believe it. But in another part of me, a small sense of fear slowly started to build up. 'Only if God wants it,' I replied to Abdel Rahman, 'the jinn only attacks if so willed by God,' part of me feeling this was an odd thing to say when really I don't believe in it, another part of me feeling a great deal of comfort and relief from having made a small *duʿāʾ*.

Real spirits exist, Turner writes. Not just as real metaphors, real concepts, or spirits that may take on a reality in a foreign ontology. They exist and are a universal part of reality, regardless of whether we believe in them or not. 'Spirit-energy is everywhere' (Turner 2006: 33).

This is the exit point, a good friend and professor at the Department of Islamic Studies told me. When you start to bring home the experiments you conduct with religious life in your fieldwork at the mosque, then it is time to end it. You have to clarify such turning points, he told me. This was five months ago, after I came home from my first real participatory encounter with the spiritual life of neo-orthodox Islam. Already at that time I thought I had to end my fieldwork; that it was going too far, I was transforming into something I could not recognise anymore. After about a week's consideration I started to calm down. Another friend and professor at the Department of Anthropology told me this is the way it is supposed to be: 'Fieldwork should transform you, otherwise you don't learn anything. Then afterwards you go to a shrink.'

I know I shouldn't bring the experiences from the mosque into my private life. Work is work. In the dark room I silently begin to recite the few phrases from the Quran I know may help protect us from the evil spirits. 'Say: I seek refuge with the Lord of mankind, the King of mankind, the God of mankind, from the evil of the whisperer who whispers evil in the hearts of men, who withdraws from his whispering in one's heart after one remembers Allah, who whispers in the breasts of mankind, of jinn and men' (Surat al-Nas 1–5).

## Notes

1 Aziz had arrived after the beginning of the *khuṭba* and started conducting the voluntary prayer for entering the mosque during the sermon of the imam.

2 Matei Candea (2011) points out how Viveiros de Castro's concept of 'seriousness' seems to divide the human race up into a sphere of intellectual debate in which there is agreement and disagreement, 'belief' and 'disbelief', and another sphere of social interaction in which there is 'taking seriously'. As Candea (2011: 148) states: 'Unlike the Amazonians, Rorty and Deleuze are not "taken seriously" – not left in a state of sustained possibility. On the contrary, Rorty's possible world is verified and rejected, just as Deleuze's possible world is verified and provides a definition of anthropology.' To be sure, taking seriously must also extend to those people who do not live within Deleuzian or multiperspectival ontologies (see also Schielke 2019).

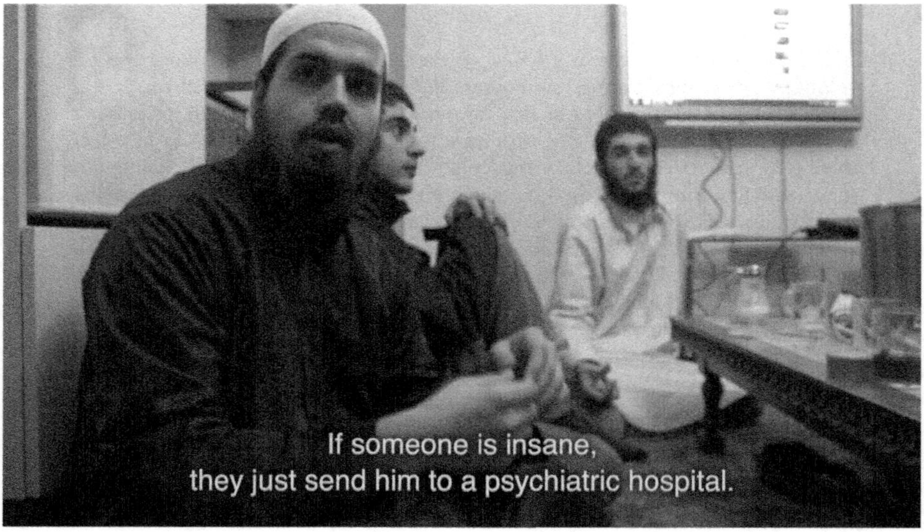


3.1 Still from Scene 7

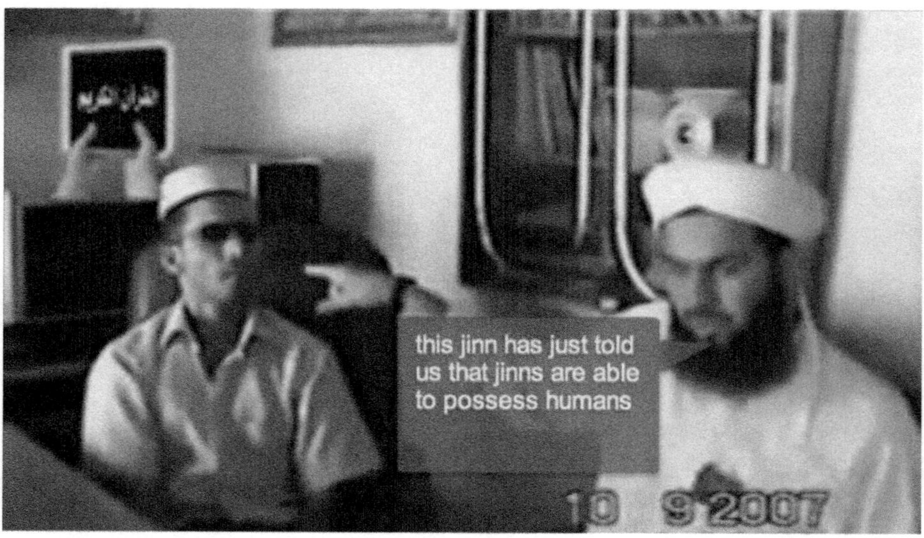
this jinn has just told
us that jinns are able
to possess humans
10 9 2007

3.2 Still from Scene 7

# 3

# Jinn exorcisms on YouTube

SEVEN young men in their late teens to early twenties sit around a coffee table with cookies, coffee, and tea in an apartment in the large social housing complex officially identified as the 'ghetto' of Gellerup, in Aarhus, Denmark. A YouTube video entitled '7000 year old jinn inside man' is playing on the large plasma TV hanging on the wall.

I became interested in this group of young Muslims when they started cleaning the garden, the party room, and the 'torture chamber' of a former biker gang club house on the outskirts of Aarhus in August 2010. The new owner, a former leader of the so-called 'immigrant gang' Black Cobra, had offered the place to the group as a way to expiate for his previous sins, which had included drug dealing, gambling, and other illegal activities.

The young men wanted to build a small mosque as a refuge from the demands of parents and the corrupting influences of Danish society. They were children of refugees or immigrants who moved to Denmark from Iraq, Lebanon, Afghanistan, Somalia, and Turkey. Some participants in the project had previously been engaged in small-scale crime, drug dealing, hash smoking, or alcohol abuse. Most of them had experienced a hard time growing up in the Danish school system. For them, neo-orthodox Islam was a way of escaping all of this, purifying their hearts, and getting their lives back on track (Suhr 2014).

I was looking forward to making an ethnographic film about their ambitious project of transforming the biker gang club house into a centre for pious Muslim youth. After five or six weeks, however, the project came to an end. Members of a neighbouring mosque had convinced the young men that it would be better to pursue their activities in an already established institution. A rift appeared between those in the group who felt that the local mosques were too limiting and politically corrupt, and those who agreed that, as young people, they still needed the advice of older generations.

In 2011, several members of the group decided to leave Denmark to study Arabic in the Middle East. It was on one such evening, gathered to say goodbye to a friend, that the talk turned to jinn possession. The young men had recently witnessed several severe cases of possession, including the possession of their friend Feisal by more than twenty-six jinn of multiple origins and religious conviction, and the possession of a young Somali boy by the Danish female jinn Dorthe, her husband, and their dog Hugin. These harrowing scenes were a favoured topic of discussion. Frequently, they would try to make sense of them by comparing their own experiences with videos on YouTube. This evening I was allowed to record their discussion.

First, we watched a video of a group of suspicious-looking shaykhs who were allegedly inserting jinn directly into their patients through the tips of their fingers. Then we saw some people identified as 'Sufis', both women and men, also apparently possessed by jinn, dancing wildly and head-banging with their robes, long beards, and hair flailing. According to the young men, practitioners of Sufism imagine that such unrestrained body movements bring them into oneness with God. The display was at once amusing and frightening: '*Aʿūdhu bi-l-Lāh*, God protect us from the Sufis ... Do you want some more coffee?'

Finally, Adrees asks the others to put on the video of the '7000 year old jinn'. The loud, determined voice of the YouTube exorcist fills the room: 'What is your religion – are you Muslim, Christian, or Jewish?'

The arms of the man possessed by the jinn move awkwardly. His head twitches to the side. The jinn stammers its answer: 'Jewish.'

The shaykh continues his inquisition in Arabic. Mubarak, who came to Denmark with his parents as a refugee from Somalia, does not speak the language. He asks Imad, who is half-Lebanese, to translate.

'[The shaykh] says: Tell us how old you are – don't lie. She says she doesn't lie. 7,000 years old.'

Adrees summarises the statements of the jinn for my camera: 'It's a female jinn called Varia. She claims that she's 7,000 years old. She's from Congo.'

Now the jinn switches to Kurdish. Imad asks Karzan, whose parents arrived in Denmark from the Kurdish part of Turkey, to translate.

Karzan is gasping at the scene: 'The jinn saw this man and she liked him. She liked him so she decided to enter him. She fell in love with this guy.'

'Does the jinn speak Kurdish?' Adrees asks. Adrees was born in Afghanistan and came to Denmark with his brother and parents as refugees. He understands some classical Arabic but not Kurdish. Chya, who sits next to Karzan and who also speaks Kurdish, confirms: 'Yes, they both speak Kurdish.'

Adrees talks to my camera again: 'This is an example: a black woman from Congo who speaks Kurdish.'

Referring to the possessed body, Imad adds: 'But he also speaks Arabic. He speaks Arabic to the camera.'

'Who is the shaykh, where is he from?' Adrees asks.

Chya replies: 'You can see he's a shaykh. At least he has left his beard.'

Imad: 'Either Kurd or Arab.'

Mubarak is getting annoyed by all the interruptions: 'Just play it.'

Adrees: 'We don't know where he's from.'

The video starts again.

Chya translates: 'Now the jinn is explaining why she possessed the man: "He was very beautiful so I chose him."'

Karzan continues the translation: 'The shaykh says, "The jinn is lying: you're lying, you don't like him." She says: "No, no, I'm not lying."'

Some of the men start to laugh. Now the voice of the shaykh is translated in green speech bubbles. He is speaking to the jinn: 'There are some people out there that do not believe that jinn can possess humans. Can a jinn possess a human?'

'Yes, yes.' The jinn confirms that this is possible.

The shaykh turns his attention to a person outside the image frame and then looks directly at the camera: 'Listen scholars, and those of you who call yourselves scholars. The jinn has just told us that jinn are able to possess humans. Witness with your own eyes on [video].'

## An example of jinn possession

Let us pause and consider this peculiar image on the TV screen (see Figure 3.2, page 54, and Scene 7).[1] A man with a thick black beard dressed in a white *jalabiyya* and a turban sits to the right of the frame. His dress and physical appearance suggest this could be a Muslim of some dedication – a shaykh perhaps, a person with religious training and authority. While looking out towards the lower left corner, perhaps speaking to a person sitting outside the frame, the shaykh points his finger directly at the face of another man behind him, to the left of the frame. This man is dressed in dark trousers and a white shirt. He is wearing a white cap of the sort many Muslims use for praying – a *taqiyya*. Sunglasses cover his eyes, but he appears to stare back at the shaykh, pointing at his face. A green speech bubble translates the shaykh's words. He is telling us that the person he is pointing at is in fact a jinn and that 'the jinn has just told us that jinn are able to possess humans'.

I have attempted to analyse the experiences and understandings my Muslims interlocutors have of jinn possession and psychosis by using the expressive qualities of both images and written text. But how do they themselves use images to understand these phenomena? And how does their use of images relate to the various ways in which images have been used in visual anthropology as a way of documenting, providing examples of, and analysing social life? Could the recurrent queries regarding the value of images in visual anthropology find new answers through exploring the responses to visual media in neo-orthodox Islam?

As Adrees points out what we are presented with is an 'example' of jinn possession – an instantiation of the type of event in which invisible spirits take residence in the visible world – in this case: 'a black woman from Congo who speaks Kurdish'. The image, in this sense, provides a case example illustrating a range of phenomena that can be grouped within the category of spirit possession. Yet as we shall see, it is a complicated case.

The image, however, is also an example in a different sense, namely in the sense of providing visual evidence for the existence of the case example – evidence of the fact that the case example as an event actually happened. The image is quite literally an imprint of the visible light and shadows that, at a specific moment, constituted this peculiar scene and were cast into and captured by the microchip of a camcorder. Through various digital translations, this mixture of light and shadow is now recast and presented to us as a sample of reality, an indexical proof of the existence of this body, which exemplifies for us how a human may become possessed by jinn.

According to the Quran and the practices and sayings of the Prophet (*sunna*), jinn exist alongside the world of humans, but the two worlds are separated (Quran 7: 27). Considerable debate persists among Islamic scholars about the possibility of jinn entering the world of humans and the extent to which they are able to do this. Within vernacular traditions, cases abound in which humans enter into alliances with these invisible creatures, even to the degree of marriage and sexual reproduction (Boddy 1989; Pandolfo 1997; Hopkins 2007; Drieskens 2008; see also Taymiyah 2007[1263–1328 C.E.]). Maarouf (2007) shows how in the maraboutic tradition he studied in Morocco, good jinn may also possess humans and how in this context possession is not by definition considered harmful (see also Khan 2006; Taneja 2017). This stands in clear contrast to the current movements of neo-orthodox Islam often identified as Salafism, in which a call is made for a return to what is considered to be the true practice of the Prophet and his immediate companions (see e.g. Sedgwick 2010). Many Muslims within these movements aim for a complete detachment from the world of jinn, as they argue that any interaction between the worlds of humans and jinn is essentially a violation of the divinely ordained decree of separation. Consequently, jinn who enter into the bodies of humans must be evil and have to either be exorcised or exterminated (Philips 2007).

The case example brought to us by YouTube in the form of a man wearing sunglasses is presented as evidence of the way in which evil jinn can enter and violate the lives of humans. Yet the example may not immediately, by its physical outline, indicate much in the way of a hostile takeover of a human body by a malicious invisible creature. A sense of confusion develops as we are watching and discussing the video – a confusion which we apparently share with many of the viewers who have left their comments. As one YouTube commenter pointed out: 'I believe in jinn … but the video is a lie a big one!!!!' Another commenter argued that '[jinn] r way 2 smart 2 let them selves be recorded … trust me 98% of the online recordings r fake … this is all just made up, not real.' As illustrated by the lengthy debate on YouTube, the case example of jinn possession is simply not enough to convince many viewers – Muslims as well as non-Muslims. For these viewers, both the possessed body and the image of the body fail to show what they were intended to exemplify.

## Salt and pepper

Adrees asks: 'Who is a Jew?'

'The jinn,' Imad replies.

Adrees is still confused: 'I thought it was from Congo?'

Imad laughs: 'Yes, but it's a Jew. It's a Jew from Congo. Congo is its nationality.'

Mubarak asks again to have the words of the jinn translated. It has shifted to Kurdish again. Its movements are becoming increasingly odd.

Chya: 'The shaykh in the video says: "I know you're not afraid of me. What is it you're afraid of?"'

Karzan takes over: 'He says: "They tell me to leave. The angels are big." He asks: "Are they larger than you?" He answers: "Yes, they're much larger than me."'

Imad has started to laugh again. Karzan continues: 'Can't we use this as evidence? She says that the angels are big and that they are present in this room. They yell and demand that it leave. So this is evidence that …'

Khalil, who has remained silent until now, interrupts: 'Evidence of what?'

'That angels exist,' Karzan replies.

Mubarak is not convinced by Karzan: 'But he says himself that jinn lie a lot.'

The discussion continues for a while and is turning into an interrogation of the truth of what is shown in the video. I speculate whether the fact that I am present with a camera adds to a degree of tension. Then the YouTube video plays again. The shaykh has started exorcising the aged Congolese jinn from the possessed man through the recitation of Surat al-Jinn (Quran 72: 1).

'Say: It has been revealed to me that a group of jinn listened to the Quran.'

This verse is often quoted as evidence of the existence of jinn as real beings who, like humans, have been endowed with the will and freedom to accept the divine message. When used in exorcism, the verse may remind the intruding jinn of how it has betrayed the law of God, but how it still has the possibility of escaping eternal torment by surrendering to the absolute deity. In this case it seems to have an effect. The possessed body is coughing loudly. The shaykh continues to recite:

'They [the jinn] said: "Verily, we have listened to a wonderful recital. It guides to the right path and we have believed therein and we shall never join anything with our Lord."'

Imad points out to us that the jinn has finally been persuaded to take the Islamic creed – *al-shahāda*: 'He testifies that there is no other god than God. He testifies that Muhammad is the messenger of God.'

Once more the jinn starts to cough. Mubarak concludes: 'Now it's leaving the body. Something is coming out of his mouth.'

The shaykh is talking in Kurdish again. Chya translates: 'He says that he has been possessed, this is evidence for those who don't believe in jinn. He's happy that he got rid of it.'

Khalil has grown increasingly sceptical during the viewing of the video: 'I don't know how many stories I have heard like this. Who knows whether they are true?'

Imad looks at him with dismay: 'You could start to believe …'

Khalil: 'Seriously, we know jinn are real – but I have heard so many stories that are totally …'

Adrees attempts to stop an argument from developing again: 'Some people tend to exaggerate. Some people like to add salt and pepper to any story that they hear.'

## The good, the bad, and the failed example

In academic discourse the word 'example' is often used to mean an attempt at illustration. The validity of the example is conceived to rest in its correspondence with reality: the degree to which it mirrors and is representative of reality (Taylor 1990: 101; Højer and Bandak 2015). When the young men discuss the possibility of using the video example as evidence of the existence of jinn and angels, it is in terms of such a correspondence: the degree to which the image and the body of the possessed faithfully mimic reality. This notion of example as illustrative or representative of reality stands in contrast to the original, but still widely used, connotation of the example as model not only *of* but also *for* the conduct of social life. An example in this older sense is not just illustrative but also morally normative by being exceptional in some way. It stands out by embodying in pure form that which it is exemplary of (Højer and Bandak 2015). In the Quran, the word *uswa* is used to describe the good example of the Prophet. Here *uswa* carries the connotation of example as a pattern to follow – or role model – *uswatun ḥasanatun*, a beautiful pattern (Quran 33: 21).

In the neo-orthodox Islamic work of faith, considerable attention is given to how one may best follow the example of the Prophet. His behaviour, manner of speech, physical appearance, and high morals are described as the finest and most perfect that has and ever will be achieved by a human. The Prophet is the embodiment of 'the good example' in the sense of being a condensation of all possible ethical values that a human being can achieve (see Robbins 2015) – the 'seal' and completion of divine prophethood. The task for the Muslim is therefore to emulate this model as best possible in all areas of life – ranging from the most trivial of everyday tasks, such as how to get up in the morning, the order in which one puts on one's shoes, and how one enters and exits a bathroom, to the important ritual procedures at birth, marriage, death, and so on (Sedgwick 2006: 9, 120).

Yet since the Prophet constitutes the asymptote of perfection, no other human can ever achieve his degree of completeness. Desires, delusional thinking, and evil forces compete tirelessly to drag ordinary humans away from this ideal example. For this reason, humans need to establish a sense of direction so they will know which way to orientate themselves. It is perhaps to this end that bad examples are also given – the worst of which is Iblis, the personification of evil in Islam. According to most Islamic scholars, Iblis was initially among the believing jinn, yet when God created humankind and asked Iblis to prostrate before Adam, he refused. From arrogance and sheer envy he turned away from God and attempted to drag humankind with him towards damnation. Since God had initially created Iblis and was therefore the master of his actions, it was also God's decision to allow Iblis's betrayal and his ever-proceeding attempts to drag believers away from the truth. In the cosmology of Islam, this primordial event marks the beginning of the divine test of humankind.

A broad continuum extends between the perfect example of goodness at one end and the ultimate example of evil at the other, as embodied by the Prophet and Iblis, respectively. Along this continuum, we find a range of examples that can be said to be neither absolutely good nor absolutely evil. Instead these examples offer a mixture of good and evil, and it is often not possible to discern whether good or evil has the upper hand. The struggle of neo-orthodox Muslims to emulate the good example of the Prophet, to become a good example for others to follow, and to turn away from the bad example of Iblis is carried out in this unknowable middle ground. It is in this intermediate region of imperfection, half-appearances, and distorted images between the visible and the invisible that most of these Muslims' lives are played out (see also Pandolfo 1997).

On this particular evening in Gellerup, the screening of the YouTube exorcism appears to ignite an unintended discussion. The video was meant to provide visual evidence of the existence of both invisible jinn and angels. As such, it was intended not so much as an example for proper Islamic conduct, but rather – as in the correspondence model in much Western social science – as a model and illustration of reality as it actually is (Schäuble 2016b: 2, 15). Instead, however, it has provoked a debate about the extent to which it is possible, necessary, or even desirable to believe in such peculiar visual displays, or whether they could in fact be make-believe on the part of either jinn, patient, shaykh, or filmmaker.

In anthropology, similar debates have occurred over the questionable value of photographic images and film in providing a window into unseen realities (Marcus 1994; Weiner 1997; MacDougall 1998; Henley 2006; Kiener 2008; Suhr and Willerslev 2012; 2013). As mentioned in Chapter 1, Hastrup (1992: 9) once attempted to photograph an Icelandic agricultural show of rams. Soon she realised that the show of rams was a secret ritual competition for male potency. Yet her photographs, in their flat two-dimensionality, were unable to convey this intense sensory experience of masculine sexuality. The deeper layers of the interaction between men and ram remained invisible to her camera.

Like our YouTube exorcism, Hastrup's failed photography seemed to point at the lack of invisibility in the visually mediated recasting of reality: look, here was the invisible, why can't we see it? Both the shaykh and Hastrup demand of the image that it shows the invisible, understood as an extraordinary realm of ritualistic, sexually charged, or magical atmosphere. Yet the problem is that the invisible cannot quite be contained within the image. Somehow the abundance of visual detail provided by the image doesn't help in grasping the traces of invisible phenomena designated by concepts such as 'jinn possession' or 'competition for male potency'. Both Hastrup and the shaykh in our YouTube video struggle to squeeze an essentially invisible phenomenon into the visible facade of an image. Their words appear better at containing the kind of invisibility that they argue persists beneath the visible facade. For Hastrup (1992: 11), her disappointing photographic experience leads to a subordination of photographic imagery as necessarily inferior to the written word in its capacity for producing anthropological knowledge. Why then do both anthropologists and pious Muslims spend their time with images if the knowledge they produce, as Hastrup (1992: 17) concludes, inevitably remains 'iconographic' and 'thin' and therefore irrelevant to any serious exploration of the unseen dimensions of human reality?

For many visual anthropologists, the issue has been not how to contain the invisible within the image, but rather how to counteract anthropology's tendency to over-amplify intangible cultural differences through excessive textual abstraction. David MacDougall points out how the visible features of human life have 'largely disappeared as signifiers of culture' (1998: 255) and how anthropology has detached itself from observable reality to such a degree that it is often impossible to discern any resemblance between lived life and the cultural formations being described. For MacDougall, the ethical potential of ethnographic film and photography lies in its way of returning us to the concrete and detailed features of persons and their environments. Visual media have, as Castaing-Taylor also argues, a capacity for exceeding theory and for 'showing anthropologists' purchase on the lived experience of their subjects to be rather more precarious than they would like to believe' (1996: 88).

At the basis of Castaing-Taylor's and MacDougall's critique of the abstractions of written anthropology is a particular understanding of how the medium of film allows us to explore the role played by ordinary lived time and space in the constitution of social life. As MacDougall argues, photographic imagery and video images have a way of inserting us into the immediacy of social life at the point at which analytical conceptions are still not fully explicated. The knowledge provided by a camera is often 'stubborn and opaque, but with a capacity for the finest detail' (MacDougall 2006: 6). Thus images allow a glimpse into a moment where thought is still undifferentiated from matter and feeling in ways that it often later loses in analytic abstractions (MacDougall (2006: 1). As MacDougall points out, photographic images and film have a way of counterbalancing the strangeness of even the most exotic people with 'a sense of familiarity' (1998: 245) – that is, a sense of how, despite cultural differences, we are ultimately all subject to the same plane of embodied spatial and temporal existence.

Both MacDougall and Castaing-Taylor are pivotal figures within the formation of observational cinema – a distinctive style of documentary filmmaking that uses the mimetic power of the camera to not simply mirror everyday reality, but facilitate a process of merging the object of perception with the body of the perceiver. Through long uninterrupted shots, the camera is used as 'a physical extension' of the cameraperson's perceptual organs, thus allowing viewers intimate access to the filmmaker's engagement with the social reality portrayed (Castaing-Taylor 1996: 75; Henley 2004: 114; Grimshaw and Ravetz 2009: 548). In this way, ethnographic filmmakers of the observational tradition seek to apply a holistic approach that avoids the fixation on verbal meaning, theoretical abstractions, and 'invisible' cultural differences in much written analysis (Grimshaw and Ravetz 2009: 539; Suhr and Willerslev 2012). Against Hastrup's critique of the incapacity of visual media to show the invisible, MacDougall (1998: 252) asks us to appreciate the image for how it shows the visible commonalities of being human, which, in his view, have disappeared from much contemporary anthropology. How do these claims for and against the image and its capacity for showing invisible realities or pan-human commonalities make sense in relation to the video of young Muslims in Gellerup watching an exorcism on YouTube?

## True or false

The YouTube video has stopped playing but the discussion continues. Just as much doubt as certainty is provoked by these images, and the scepticism aroused does not confine itself to the space of the image, but spills over to other instances of possession that the young men have witnessed or heard about.

Khalil asks: 'Why believe it, you don't know if it's real?'

Imad: 'If there are witnesses.'

Khalil: 'It could be true but it could also be false.'

Chya: 'Don't you believe your brother?' Chya refers to the previous discussion about two cases of possession that some of the members of the group have personally witnessed.

Khalil: 'He has experienced something. I'm not saying it's untrue. But many of the examples we have talked about ...'

Imad interrupts: 'If, for example, I tell you that I have seen all this with our Bosnian brother, would you trust me? Yes, because I have experienced it myself.'

Khalil replies: 'Yes, you have seen it, but when I hear a story that someone has heard from another – I can't use it for anything. Why should I care?'

Adrees tries again to end the argument: 'I do understand you. You can never use such a story as evidence. Evidence of what is allowed and what is forbidden. But such stories can awaken you – awaken your seriousness. They teach us that we have to protect ourselves – from evil spirits and magic – by reading those verses that the Prophet, peace be upon him, has taught us. It's good if we read them.'

Khalil, still not satisfied: 'Just before, I heard this story. He said that the trees could move during the night and that they could enter into the rectum of some animal ... I don't have this from the Quran or the *Sunna*. Why should I accept it?'

Again Adrees makes an effort to settle the discussion: 'But in any case ... the conclusion of this is that such stories are not obligatory for you to believe in. It's not demanded of you to believe in them. But what you and all Muslims have to believe is what the Prophet, peace be upon him, has said. For example, the Prophet said that the jinn can fly. Then we believe it. Okay, this is possible for jinn. But if we hear some other story, then you can question it. Okay, maybe I believe this story or I don't believe it – because the storyteller is a liar or something else. But I believe that a jinn can fly. That this is possible. I just don't know if this particular story is true. Like with any other story – who tells it? Who has witnessed the story? Does the story seem realistic?'

## The limits of perception

Somehow the reality depicted by the YouTube video appeared to fall apart as we watched it. The video showed precisely how to get rid of jinn by reading the Quran, how a dark magical substance was thrown up at the climax of the exorcism, and how finally the human subject repossessed his body. Nevertheless, the video showed so much that the event almost took on the appearance of a parody. Some of the young men were from the outset of the discussion inclined to appreciate the video as evidence of the miracle of the Quran while others reacted sceptically, but as the conversation continued it was clear that no one had their presuppositions fully affirmed.

At the moment of filming, I attempted – in the style of observational cinema – to let the camera blend in and not unnecessarily intrude in the unfolding of the discussion. Obviously, however, the presence of the camera had an impact on the discussion. The declared aim of the young Muslims is to be as best they can 'the face of the Prophet of God in Denmark'. However, in this case, the camera as witness to their embodiment of divinely ordained conduct intensified the discussion so that what was intended as an exemplification of the truth of God ended up as a rather muddled conversation about falsity and mischief.

The most basic demand on the neo-orthodox Muslim is to bear witness to the existence of the invisible domain of God, paradise, hell, angels, and jinn (Quran 2: 2–5). The religious duty, however, is not simply to take at face value any visual illustration of the invisible. In fact, many of the Muslims I worked with stated that any attempt at visualising the invisible was not only impossible but also forbidden (see also Wahhab 1996[1703–1792 C.E.]: 174). As Abu Bilal argued, there would be no meaning to faith, testimony, or God's test of humankind if people could already see the invisible (*al-ghayb*).

The invisible, as understood in the context of neo-orthodox Islam, is precisely that which cannot be reached through the senses. Hence it is not a job for human beings to attempt to do this. But when the invisible appears to intrude into the visible world, it is difficult to know how one should react. In this case, the visual display of the invisible divided the participants in the discussion. While some, like the shaykh in the YouTube video, strived to claim the image as an evidential example of the existence of jinn, and therefore a platform upon which they could testify to divine truth, others in the discussion felt obliged to react with scepticism at the visualisation of the invisible.

Several of the young men found themselves incapable of not bursting into laughter as they witnessed the scene. For them, perhaps in a similar way as for filmmakers and visual anthropologists of the observational tradition, the visual display pointed towards a more 'ordinary' reality, standing in marked contrast to the extraordinary verbal claims of the shaykh. In MacDougall's (1998: 250) view the 'ordinary' signifies human commonalities that radically transcend the cultural difference invoked in much written anthropology. For the young Muslims, however, the ordinary is also the realm of pretend and make-believe, which, in their view, has become increasingly dominant in modern society.

When I watch these film examples of young pious Muslims watching exorcisms, I am not at all sure whether it leads me to a recognition of radical impermeable difference or more ordinary human commonalities. Rather, what it leaves me with is confusion. By no means does it display the kind of fullness and homogeneity of space and time favoured by observational filmmakers. Instead, the observational scene seems to shuffle indistinctly between the actual and virtual, between past, present, and future. This heterogeneous meshwork issues from the co-presence of multiple realities, temporalities, objects, appearances, and voices that completely exceed the limited space and temporality of the film-image. I simply do not know where to situate the 'normal human participant' (Henley 2004: 114) who allegedly has the capacity of a pan-human perception in this setting. Could this be me as the camera operator? Is it the shaykh? Is it the possessed? The jinn? Is it those young men who cannot see or believe in the evidential proof presented to us? Or is it those who do see and believe in it? If there is an element of pan-human perception that we share in this conglomerate of vision, then it can only be located in the failure of perception and in the situatedness and obvious limitation of human perception.

## Exorcising humility

Hirschkind points out how Muslim YouTube-surfing of this kind can best be described as an adventure 'across a quixotic, unpredictable landscape whose every twist and turn presents not the threads of an unfolding discourse or the development of a deeper understanding but the sudden surprise of an affect, the pleasure or shock of an unexpected discovery' (2012: 5). Hirschkind is primarily exploring the practice of watching sermons (*khuṭub*) on YouTube. Based on the comments left by Muslim viewers, he concludes that the prime attraction of such videos is their capacity to move the viewer towards experiences of pious tranquillity (*iṭmi'nān*), stillness of the soul (*sakīna*), and humility (*khushū'*). Videos that arouse the heart towards such ethical and devotional dispositions are frequently described as *mu'aththir* – a term indicating that something is effective, moving, or exciting (Hirschkind 2012: 6). Muslim YouTube viewers often leave comments in the form of small supplications (*du'ā'*) – a kind of visual and ethical testament to repeated acts of drawing close to God. However, according to Hirschkind, the moral space that is created by these commentaries is highly vulnerable. If YouTube viewers leave derogatory comments, the effectiveness of the videos in arousing the correct emotional response seems to dramatically decrease.

Hirschkind (2012: 13) analyses the use of *khuṭba*-videos as well as videos of beautiful babies and awe-inspiring natural phenomena, all of which could be said to embody good examples in the sense of constituting 'modest images'. By contrast, I draw attention here to videos that are very difficult to think of as good examples, yet still produce a kind of shock that attracts pious Muslim youth. When watching these exorcisms, the shock of the image provokes amazement and wonder, but also a kind of rib-tickling entertainment verging on the inappropriate. The comical and the potentially inappropriate do not appear, however, to distract Muslim viewers from the videos. Despite highly disparaging comments about 'barbaric Arabs' or the 'backwardness' of Islam, large numbers of viewers continue to watch, comment, and copy '7000 year old jinn inside man'. Somehow, the capacity of these rather immodest, failed images to arouse a devotional response is not as easily polluted as the YouTube sermons analysed by Hirschkind. In fact, it seems that accusations of falsity as well as anti-Islamic comments left by non-Muslims stimulate the popularity of and debate around these videos of exorcism on YouTube. How can we make sense of this?

The notion of an audio-visual 'shock' used by Hirschkind to describe the experience offered to pious Muslims by YouTube brings to mind a style of filmmaking very different from the realist schools discussed so far in this chapter. Most ethnographic filmmakers in the observational tradition have been preoccupied with the 'cinema of duration' as advocated by André Bazin (2005[1967]: 39; Grimshaw and Ravetz 2009: 539) – that is, the ability of the camera to capture events and actions in human life in the order and pace in which they actually occur. Rather than shocking the viewer, the aim is to allow the viewer to become immersed in the observation of a single moment in a particular place. In contrast, the early Soviet cinema of filmmakers such as Sergei Eisenstein and Dziga Vertov was aimed precisely at producing cinematic shocks.

In Eisenstein's (1949) conception, 'intellectual montage' as opposed to 'mundane montage' referred to a juxtaposition of dissimilar objects which, when put in confrontation with each other, would shock the viewer into recognising a reality far larger than could possibly be seen from a single subjective viewpoint. Rather than aligning viewers with a certain reality, Eisenstein saw in cinema the essential tools for people to stand up to oppressive ideas of what counts as the real. In his words: 'The representation of objects in the actual (absolute) proportions proper to them is, of course, merely a tribute to orthodox formal logic … [d]isplacing the expressiveness of archaic disproportion for regulated "stone tables" of officially decreed harmony' (Eisenstein 1949: 34–5).

By contrast, the cinema of montage implied an aesthetics where each juxtaposition of film shots constituted a qualitative leap out of the perceptual regimes that dominate human action and thought (see also Deleuze

2005a[1986]: 38). Instead of the correspondence model of observational cinema, the filmmaking pursued by early Soviet filmmakers aimed at the transgression of the observable. Here validity was to be measured not by the resemblance of a film to the 'pro-filmic', but rather by its power to force the viewer out of the pro-filmic and into empathy and passionate engagement in the joint production of an industrial communist utopia (see e.g. Vertov 1929).

Can contemporary neo-orthodox Muslim YouTube viewing be understood as a consumption of images akin to that imagined by Eisenstein and Vertov? In exposing themselves to videos such as '7000 year old jinn inside man', these young Muslim men are not uniting their perception with that of a camera. Rather, the juxtaposition of elements internal to this video, to other videos, and to the experiences and comments of other viewers creates fissures that force the pro-filmic display outside of itself. The odd character of the display, the bird's-eye view camera, the bold postulates of the shaykh, the strange discontinuous YouTube subtitling, and the harsh debate left by hundreds of viewers all work to forge cracks in the visible facade. For Eisenstein, the perceptual disruptions facilitated by cinema were necessary for the emergence of the communist paradise. Are Muslim YouTube viewers using these videos in a similar way, as a vehicle to enhance the ethical conduct and sensitivity required for entering the Gardens of Everlasting Bliss (Quran 9: 72)?

Surely part of the attraction for the group of young Muslims in viewing exorcisms of jinn is entertainment. Yet it is not only entertainment. The excitement and horror of viewing these videos stems from the small gaps of ontological insecurity that are produced. For pious Muslims, these cracks into the unknown may be useful because they produce a degree of doubt. Doubt (*shakk*) is often described as one of the most dangerous forms of illness. Yet doubt is an unavoidable condition and perhaps, in fact, a necessity. Without doubt, there would be complete certainty and therefore no possibility of faith as an active submission of consciousness to the divine. The emphasis on such paradoxical movements of faith is present in a number of religious traditions within and beyond Islam. Kierkegaard, whose translated work is being used by a number of Islamic scholars, argued, for example, that doubt is indeed the very engine of faith (Kierkegaard 2005[1843]; see Bektovic 1999; Kassim 1971; Tomlinson 2014).

By being exposed to '7000 year old jinn inside man', the consciousness and analytical capacity of the Muslim viewer is stretched to accommodate degrees of both belief and unbelief. Combining belief with unbelief is dangerous within neo-orthodox Islam. How can one know whether one is laughing at the individual case example or at the more general use of the Quran to exorcise spirits as it was practised and advocated by the Prophet? The latter is, in the understanding of these Muslims, tantamount to expelling oneself from the people of paradise (*ahl al-janna*). As a shaykh explained to some of the young men during their weekly lecture in basic Islamic doctrines (*'aqīda*), laughing at or in any way ridiculing the practices of the Prophet is one of the greatest sins. The enforced stretching of consciousness between belief and unbelief is not so far from the most dangerous illness of all – namely, the illness of *nifāq*: hypocrisy or double dealing. It is said that *al-munāfiq*, the hypocrite, is the person who gets the lowest position in hell. Ordinary heathens will be standing with their feet on the heads of *al-munāfiqūn*. To enter the territory between belief and unbelief is to also consequently enter a limbo between prospects for eternal life in paradise and an eternity at the very bottom of hell.

The intention with the YouTube video discussed here is that it should work as an example in the Geertzian sense – as a model of and a model for the practice of *ruqya*. For some it may work in this way. Yet because of its peculiar visual facade, it also provokes a different form of religiosity, perhaps more akin to the form of humility that may arise when encountering phenomena such as a storm or a weird dream (Schilbrack 2005: 430), and hence the kind of devotion, submission, pleas for help, or thankfulness that arises when standing before the totally invisible. It is dangerous to laugh at practices that could be of prophetic origin, or to claim to be able to identify the visible form of something invisible, but reactions like this are almost unavoidable when viewing such videos as '7000 year old jinn inside man'. In this way, the obscurity of the video pushes moral imagination and perception to their limits. While a genuinely 'good example' that is both a model *of* and a model *for* may create a path and direction for human agency, these failed images give no clear direction. Rather, they seem to dismantle the capacity for human action. Instead of devices for producing clarity or evidence, these failed images work as amplifiers of invisibility.

'It gives us a way to remember to read our daily prayers', Adrees concludes, after deciding that '7000 year old jinn inside man' cannot, after all, be taken as indisputable evidence of the divine truth. While some of the young men initially appeared convinced and argued for the truth-value of the YouTube exorcism as others fiercely argued against it, this synthesis proposed by Adrees is what they all finally agree on. If the proposed visual evidence only testifies to the fact that ultimately there is no tangible evidence, then what it provides instead is a test of one's trust in God – *al-tawakkul 'alā Allāh* – and a test of one's willingness to surrender all scepticism to the fact that the invisible is invisible and therefore cannot be seen. By collapsing the possibility of coherent signification, the failed image flows with ambiguity – speaking to its recipient from no single identifiable position. This is the curse of the image, but also its attraction and marvel, since the failure creates an ideal condition for leaps of faith, submission, and surrendering of the self to the unknown. I suggest that in this way, these odd videos become productive as a means of establishing the attitude of humility (*khushū'*) that Hirschkind points out is so pivotal in the practice of Muslim YouTube consumption.

## Images in anthropology

In what way may YouTube videos such as '7000 year old jinn inside man' help us in the anthropological pursuit of taking other people's realities seriously? What may such YouTube videos teach us with regard to the use of photographic imagery and video in anthropology? Apparently images do not work well in visually exemplifying for us the kinds of textual invisibility of which Hastrup writes. Nor do they show us in any clear-cut way the pan-human commonalities proposed by ethnographic filmmakers of the observational tradition. My argument so far can be summarised by the statement that for all their failure and incompleteness, images as examples may still be productive in establishing the possibility of a stance of humility and an appreciation of the invisible as invisible: that is, as something that cannot be seen from the perspective of a human.

In making this argument I have emphasised the ways in which the disruptive qualities of these YouTube videos parallel in certain respects the work of montage propagated by Eisenstein and Vertov. Nonetheless there are also clear differences we need to attend to.

For many viewers the invisible was not made visible in the YouTube video discussed despite the emphatic attempts of the shaykh. By contrast, both Eisenstein and Vertov found the tools to actually see into the invisible through cinematic montage, to see not only the gross exploitation of the working class by the bourgeoisie occurring right beneath the surfaces of social interaction but also the alternative futures of a harmonious communist society. As Walter Benjamin (1968) famously described, filmmaking works in this way like a surgical operation. The filmmaker penetrates the web of reality like a surgeon cutting into the body of a patient. In Benjamin's (1968: 234) words, 'the representation of reality by the film is [a] thoroughgoing permeation of reality with mechanical equipment' whereby 'multiple fragments … are assembled under a new law'. Vertov exemplified this view of filmmaking in his proposal for the new electric man: 'I am kino-eye. From one person I take the hands, the strongest and most dexterous; from another I take the legs, the swiftest and most shapely; from a third, the most beautiful and expressive head – and through montage I create a new, perfect man' (Vertov 1984: 17).

Eisenstein and Vertov's films – most notably perhaps *Man with a Movie Camera* (Vertov 1929) – were essentially constructivist, in the sense that the truth and the new vision they produced were a possibility of seeing, and thereby creating, the splendour of the young post-revolutionary communist society as a whole organic body of humans and machines moving forward in symbiosis. For my interlocutors, however, there can be no such utopian realisation in this earthly world. The invisible is invisible, and the future – paradise as well as hell – will first be seen in the afterlife. The disturbances and 'montage shocks' provided by the YouTube videos do not result in full revelation. On the contrary, they work to enfold the viewing subject in even further coils of invisibility. While Eisenstein and Vertov's methods of montage are helpful for developing an understanding of the shock effects of these YouTube videos, we need to look elsewhere to understand what happens in the vacuum of visibility that emerges beyond shock.

In visual anthropology, many filmmakers emphasise the virtues of careful observation. Here the image is often appreciated for its mimetic, indexical realism, and for the way it shows us an abundance of visual details that are often otherwise left unnoticed. Yet several filmmakers and scholars have criticised this realist approach as an ocular-centric obsession with visuality characteristic of the 'modern enlightened West'. As Laura U. Marks (2000: 133) describes, this 'critique asserts that ethnographic photography and film have objectified non-Western cultures and made a spectacle of them; they have reduced cultures to their visual appearance; and they have used vision as part of a general will to knowledge of the other as a means to power'. While not seeking to condemn vision as such, Marks (2000: 129) highlights the work of a number of recent filmmakers who counter the primacy of vision through disruptive and what she calls 'haptic' techniques that blur the possibility of full identification and leave the viewer in the realm of the inexpressible.

One such filmmaker is Trinh T. Minh-ha. In criticising the aesthetics of much realist ethnographic filmmaking devoted to long observational takes, wide-angle shots, and maximal depth of field, Trinh (1991: 53) explores the ambiguous and creative potential of the intervals occurring in rapid transitions and juxtapositions between images, words, and sounds. Her controversial film *Reassemblage* (1982) is perhaps the most vivid example. Using audio-video de-synchronisation, along with continuous abrupt jump-cuts of Senegalese women breastfeeding their babies, crying or laughing children, traditional dancing, and corn-grinding, the film directs the attention of viewers outside the screen and towards their own acts of seeing and the ways in which ethnographic films conventionally establish their subjects. In this way, the film-image leaves the regime of ocular mastery and becomes what Deleuze (2005b: 127) calls a 'power of the false' (see also Taussig 1999; Marks 2000: 65). It pushes the viewer into a crisis of truth, or as Trinh (1991: 145) phrases it, a kind of unknowable limitless field.

While clearly not intended as a forgery or deflation of truth, '7000 year old jinn inside man' can be seen as performing exactly this. Formally the composition of this video seems to have little in common with the rapid montage characteristic of Trinh's or Vertov's work. In fact it consists entirely of long observational tripod shots, quite similar to the now discarded mode of hyper-empiricist 'fly-on-the-wall' filmmaking advocated by Margaret Mead (see e.g. Bateson and Mead 1952; Mead and Bateson 1977). Yet the long observational shots of the YouTube video are forgers of a kind, or what in Deleuze's (2005b: 124) vocabulary could be called 'false continuity shot[s]'. The video is intended to provide the undeniable ground of evidence in order for judgement to be made. But in attempting this in such a decisive and unambiguous way, it effectively suspends the possibility of judgement. The longer the shot, the greater the disruptive effect. In a roundabout and perhaps accidental way, the failed image comes to share a similarity with the kind of 'ethical writing' that philosophers such as Levinas and Maurice Blanchot associate with forms of poetry that bespeak the unknown. In Blanchot's words:

> To speak the unknown, to receive it through speech while leaving it unknown, is precisely not to take hold of it, not to comprehend it; it is rather to refuse to identify it even by sight ... To live with the unknown before one ... is to enter into the responsibility of a speech that speaks without exercising any form of power. (1993[1969]: 302)

For Levinas and Blanchot, to encounter the failed image is the potentially traumatic exposure of oneself to the unknown other. It is a confrontation of the self with an alterity that cannot be grasped in any definite form (Bankovsky 2004). The image, in this sense, becomes not a looking-glass to or representation of another world; rather, in the words of Gerald A. Bruns, it becomes 'the materialization of being, the way a cadaver is the image of the deceased, a remainder or material excess of being ... not a reproduction of a thing but ... a withdrawal of it' (2006: 215). By blocking consciousness, the failed image disables the possibility of meaning, of turning the world into a symbol. As Levinas points out, the failed image does not 'extend between us and a reality to be captured'. Instead, as a 'symbol in reverse', it pushes us to an ontological dimension outside the order of the visible (Levinas 1987b: 5–7).

If we cannot fully appreciate the image for what it succeeds in depicting, then I propose, following Levinas and Blanchot, that we appreciate it for what it fails to depict. What is interesting about the video image discussed in this article is not primarily its actual visible content. Just as interesting is what it fails to show: that is, the invisible parts of reality that it brings to our attention. In some way, all images evoke the invisible simply by their framing, their carving out of a certain space, their limited range of contrast, colour reproduction, and delimitation of a certain period of time. Chained as it is to the messy and disturbing particularities of life, the image captured by a camcorder or a camera is, almost by default, exemplary in the negative – always capturing a little too little and a little too much. For Roland Barthes (2010[1980]), this photographic viewing experience of a lack and a surplus is captured by the notion of 'punctum' – often described as the visual detail that somehow constantly drags the eye outside the frame towards an invisible excess of untamed, unanalysed, perplexing life. This is also what Castaing-Taylor (1996: 76) points to when arguing how, rather than reducing people's lives to abstract analytical categories, the shots of a camera drag us into the 'ambiguity of meaning that is at the heart of human experience itself'.

## Possessed by the visible

In this chapter I have speculated upon a particular video image depicting an instance of jinn possession. Visually extreme manifestations of spirit possession have long captured the minds of ethnographic and documentary filmmakers (see e.g. Rouch 1955; Connor, Asch, and Asch 1980; Deren 1985; Vachani 1990; Herzog 1993; Aaltonen 2001; Kildea and Simon 2005; Behrend, Dreschke, and Zillinger 2015). Perhaps a part of the uncanny attraction of these phenomena lies in the way in which their visual display evokes a broader experience of possession: namely, the way in which human vision itself is possessed by the visible.

In Levinas's (1987b: 118) formulation, 'sight is … an openness and a consciousness, [and] even in its subordination to cognition, sight maintains contact and proximity. The visible caresses the eye. One sees and one hears like one touches'. This tactility of vision is further described by Marks (2000: 133) as the haptic experience that may arise when the relationship between vision and knowledge is troubled. However, in this notion of sight as the visible's caress of the eye, a certain passivity on the part of the beholder is also emphasised (see Deleuze 2005b: 124). The pre-subjective and invisible origin of vision has been thoroughly described by Merleau-Ponty (2002), who makes clear how any actual subjective visual experience is dependent on its being seen from an infinitely vast network of viewpoints – an anonymous seeing which is always already in place, waiting to inscribe the perceiving subject within it (see Kelly 2005; Suhr and Willerslev 2012). Perhaps vision in Levinas's sense – as the effect of the visible's caress – is too weak a concept, however. At least we may note how, at times, we feel exposed to a form of unwanted caress – a violence of sorts – from which we may attempt to find shelter by closing our eyes. This defence is only frail, however. Having first intruded into the retina, the visible continues to work in our imagination regardless of whether we want it to or not. As a wanted or unwanted gift, the visible transforms us in ways we cannot possibly master or repay. The primordial indebtedness of vision is impressed on us by the visual display of spirit possession and the photographic image, which is always and necessarily possessed by what it depicts.

Sometimes our ability to move around with our gaze – to select that which we wish to look at or to close our eyes – results in a common-sense understanding of vision as centred upon the perceiver. The wide array of cinematic manipulations available to the film editor also conjures this illusion of optical mastery. It is exactly this that is brought into question by the tension and limited visual display of the possessed image. Just as the body in the image is allegedly possessed by a jinn, so the image itself is possessed by the figure of two men, someone outside the frame to whom they are speaking, a physical space, and an observing camera – all of which extends beyond what can possibly be contained within the image, yet determines how we can see the image and our options with it. The failed image serves here as a warning against the clarity and security we may feel through the use of seemingly 'good' examples that too easily confirm preconceived understandings of the immediately visible. The power of visual exemplification lies not only in what an image shows, but in the incompleteness and failure of the image, its manner of 'punctum', the way in which it does not quite signify that which it appears to record: the way it leads us outside the frame.

In this book and film about psychiatric and Islamic healing, I have tried to take the 'non-representability' of image and text as a virtue (see also Trinh 1991; Suhr and Willerslev 2012). Yet in the production of both text and film, new forms of visuality and conceptual grasp are constantly forming and I am often unsure which directions these forms are taking me in. What lies on the other side of the disruptive deconstruction facilitated by montage? For some filmmakers and theoreticians it is the promise of a kind of limitless becoming, in which judgement has been suspended and the boundaries between self and other have lost their power to restrain. Indeed, for Deleuze (2005b: 142), it is the birth of human creativity.

If we can conceive of Islamic YouTube consumption in terms of such disruptive film aesthetics, then it must be emphasised that for the Muslim YouTube viewers, the disruptions facilitated by these videos are not at all to be compared with the setting free of the human spirit proposed by postmodern filmmakers and theoreticians. Rather, this disturbance facilitates a resubmission to an invisible whole, namely the law of God (see also Marks 2010: 12, 47). Thus in this case the suspension of one's own power of judgement leads to the wholehearted embrace of a divinely ordained system of judgement. The frailty and even dissolution of the subject in the face of the invisible described by philosophers such as Merleau-Ponty, Levinas, and Deleuze has much in common with Islamic understandings of the contingent character of human existence. Yet for my interlocutors realising this does not evoke any form of pure limitless becoming. Quite simply, it evokes a return to God.

If my film and book are to some extent seeking to apply the powerful tools of disruptive montage, then I need to consider what sort of totality or reassembling could take place on the other side. The claim shared by Merleau-Ponty and Levinas – that the visible only obtains its visibility on account of its insertion into a wider ground of infinite invisibility – may seem somewhat paradoxical. If we accept it, it should be possible to claim the opposite as well – namely, that by the same token the perception of the invisible as invisibility is dependent on the visible. Just as we need the invisible in order to see the visible, so is the visible a necessary requirement for evoking the invisible. This is what Merleau-Ponty (1997: 142; Dillon 1983) points to with the so-called 'reversibility thesis' – an attempt to counter the dualist distinction between objects and subjects in much Western philosophy. According to Merleau-Ponty, rather than such a radical bifurcation between consciousness and inanimate substance, what characterises human existence is a state of mutual dependency. Perceiving the other is, in other words, simultaneously also the realisation that the other perceives me. Yet even though the other's seeing me is the necessary background for my own seeing, the way the other sees me is necessarily invisible to me. As M. C. Dillon (1983: 377) argues, to see the other's seeing me 'would entail living his body while, at the same time, retaining my own incarnate being, i.e., it would entail being his body while still being mine'. For Merleau-Ponty such an all-encompassing and (at least from a human standpoint) inaccessible vision can only be made present through a kind of imagination that takes as its starting point the inadequacy of our actual perception.

The consumption of failed images and the witnessing of possessed bodies by young neo-orthodox Muslims might be one such strategy to make the invisible present through a failed visualisation. But what about the exorcist in the video? How are we to understand his behaviour? What can we conclude about him from the almost grotesque display of certainty that he conjures through his words and physical demeanour? Is he the only one who has not understood the inevitable failure of such a hopeless project of visualising the invisible? Or is he in fact able to see through the visible facade of the world to a realm hidden from the sight of the sceptical YouTube viewer?

Both the Muslim healers as well as the psychiatrists and nurses I worked with oscillate between statements of doubt, disbelief, and absolute certitude in their engagement with the invisible interior of their patients. In the act of healing, these healers expose degrees of certitude that parallel that of the YouTube shaykh, yet when they are approached outside the actual healing encounter, doubts and uncertainties very quickly appear to sneak in. In what follows I shall suggest that this oscillation is a crucial element in the transformation of persons into patients.

## Notes

1 The video entitled '7000 year old jinn inside man', with English subtitles, was originally accessed on YouTube on 14 May 2012 at www.YouTube.com/watch?v=mo1WfroDCVc. Since 2012 the video has been reposted and debated on various other channels with different titles, including 'Real jin 7000 years old': www.youtube.com/watch?v=p42lyC5ZCls and 'Shoking 7000 year old jinn inside man': www.youtube.com/watch?v=wowGQ6DR7jQ. See also Suhr 2015.

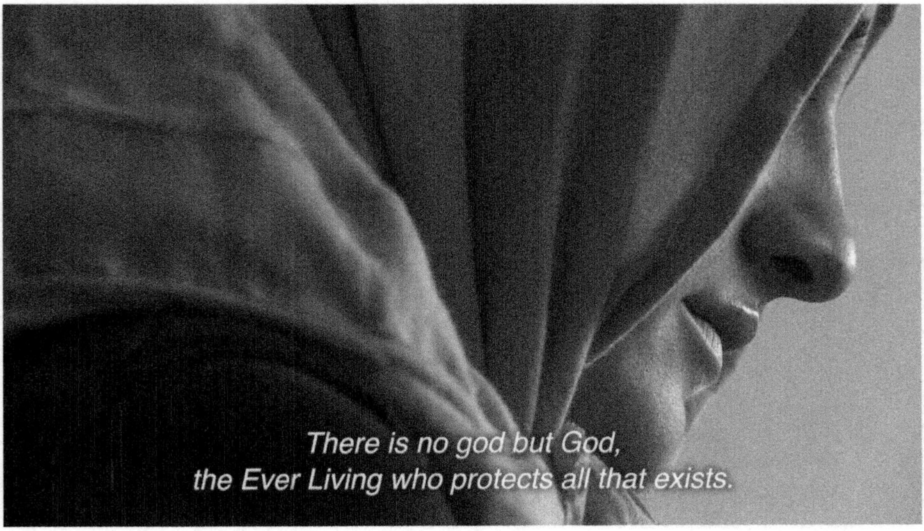
There is no god but God,
the Ever Living who protects all that exists.

4.1 Still from Scene 5

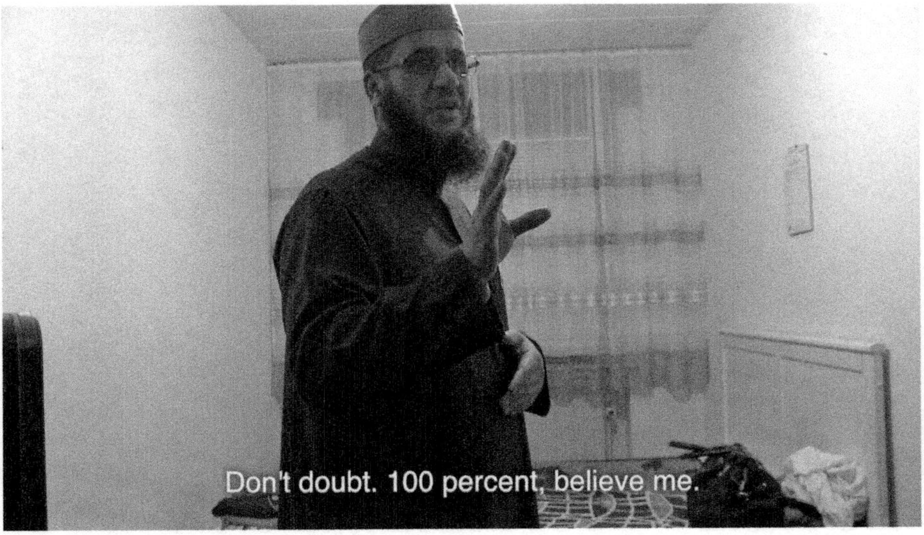
Don't doubt. 100 percent, believe me.

4.2 Still from Scene 5

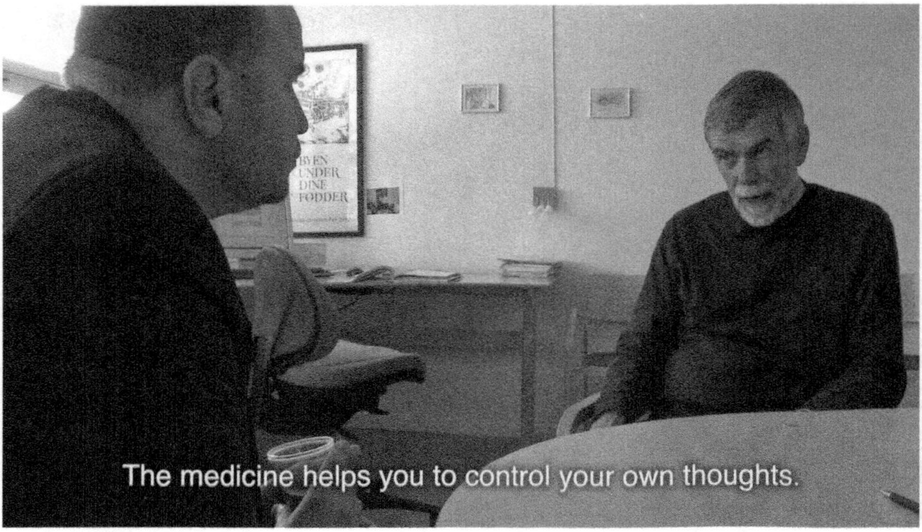


4.3 Still from Scene 4

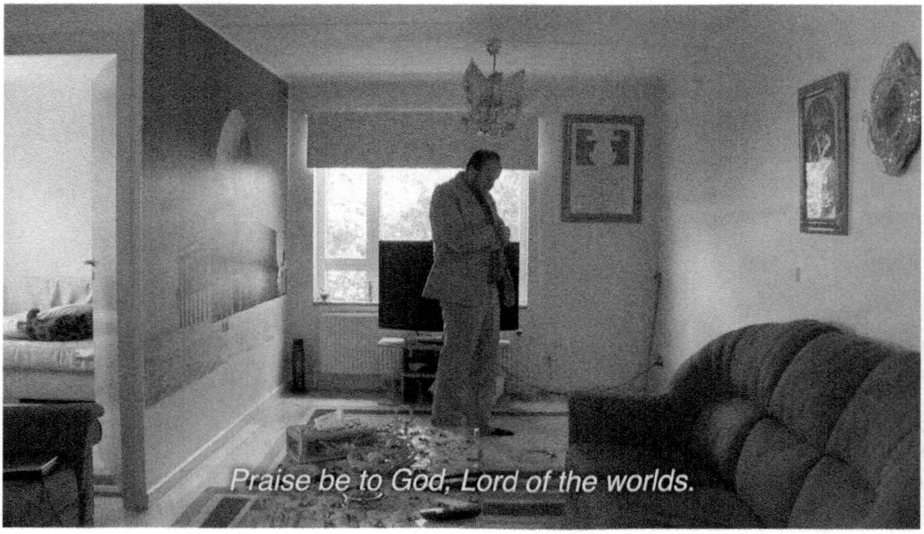


4.4 Still from Scene 3

4

# How to become a patient

THE term *ṣarʿ* designates the state a person enters when consciousness is lost and the jinn takes over full control of the body. It is derived from the verb *ṣaraʿa*, meaning to strike down or bring to the ground. In modern Arabic the term is also used to describe epilepsy. *Ṣarʿ* may be provoked by Quranic readings (*ruqya*) that force the jinn to identify itself – literally by burning the jinn so that the pain it suffers within the human body becomes manifest. However, this unconscious state may also erupt without direct provocation of the jinn.[1]

The first time I saw Feisal entering *ṣarʿ* was after a dawn prayer (*ṣalāt al-fajr*) in early 2011. At this point it was as if instances of jinn possession were breaking out almost everywhere around me. When I began this research project in 2009, I could hardly get anyone to talk about possession. Jinn possession, people told me, is something that occurs only in the Middle East. Jinn do not live in Europe. I should go back to Egypt to conduct this research as there I would find lots of this stuff, and magic, and people who understand how to deal with it. Here in Denmark it is not like this.

In 2011 I was barely able to talk to a person without being presented with a new story about someone being or having been possessed, attacked by magic, or inflicted by the evil eye at some point in their lives. This had to do partly with me having decided or accepted to take on some of the Islamic practices of worship. A couple of times I broke down in overwhelming experiences during prayer. The people in the mosque continually emphasised that my tears were an expression of *khushūʿ* – a humbling and softening of my heart – and that I should be grateful that God had allowed this to happen to me. By regularly taking part in prayer, conducting ritual ablutions, and visibly being touched by the angels and the Quranic recitation, I became for my interlocutors a testimony of divine truth. Also my frequent expressions of doubt and frustration about being split between actively taking part in Islamic practices of worship while still living a very Danish, secular life and not being able to fulfil the normative demands of either of these modes of existence seemed to testify to the truth of God. People could see in me the battle between good and evil taking place. As they explained, the moment a person decides to take up prayer is the moment they are attacked most intensely by the whispering of *shayāṭīn* – evil jinn and humans. Their retelling of their own or other people's experiences of clashes with jinn became part of their attempts to help me onto the straight path (*al-ṣirāṭ al-mustaqīm*).

But sometimes I got the feeling that my presence and interest in jinn were perhaps even attracting or accelerating the instances of jinn possession taking place around me. It is common knowledge that when you talk about jinn they become interested, as if you open a door to them (see e.g. Drieskens 2008: 50). But it is also common knowledge that anthropologists tend to overrate the impact they have on the communities they study. So much more is going on in people's lives that is of greater importance than talking to the anthropologist. Ultimately, even though our presence, participation, interviewing, and observations as anthropologists always and unavoidably alter the object of study and become part of its internal dynamics, the impact may not be as significant as we sometimes think (see e.g. Otto 1997: 96; Metcalf 2002: 45). In any case, there seemed to be an increased frequency of jinn possession in the first half of 2011. Several of the young mosque attendants also expressed surprise, as they had never seen a possession themselves.

I had first heard about Feisal during Ramadan in August 2010. I had met Adrees and some of his friends who frequented a neighbouring, competing neo-orthodox mosque. They told me about a highly disturbing event that had taken place during evening prayer (*ṣalāt al-maghrib*) a few weeks earlier. When a visiting shaykh from Egypt had started reciting the Quran, Feisal had been paralysed. Everyone in the mosque had gathered around him and the shaykh had continued to recite the Quran over him. After a while, to the great astonishment of the gathered crowd, Feisal's body had started to levitate from the ground.

Having heard this story, I became interested in finding out what was going on at this mosque. Some of Feisal's friends tried to help me get in touch with him, but he refused to meet me. Later that year I heard the story from one of the shaykhs who had participated in the exorcism of Feisal. I had been allowed to join in an exorcism of the brother of my Somali friend Abdel Rahman. Abdel Rahman wanted to bring along a proper shaykh, but unfortunately no one seemed to have time. Abdel Rahman decided to carry out the exorcism himself, since he had tried once before to exorcise his sister's jinn with some success. Before the exorcism he sought the guidance of the shaykh who had exorcised Feisal.

'You have to be strong, you must not be afraid, they'll feel this, and then they'll use you. They use your fear.'

Never to fear the jinn was the primary advice of the shaykh. He exemplified this with the story of Feisal, whose jinn had apparently become truly afraid: 'With Feisal, he still doesn't dare to look at me. There still is someone in him, I know it, he sits in his leg, Marco is his name. Feisal walks badly because of it.'

The shaykh explained how the jinn flow in the blood of the possessed and how Feisal at the time had been possessed by a great number of them. He confirmed that Feisal had actually levitated the first time they exorcised him. Jinn, especially of Jewish origin, often have the capacity to fly. The shaykh also told of some of the other jinn who had been exorcised from Feisal on subsequent occasions. Maria had been an especially entertaining experience: 'When she was in him she batted the eyelashes and tried to sweet-talk and seduce me.'

Malek, however, had been the strongest of the jinn. When they finally succeeded in converting him to Islam, he started to throw out the remaining jinn in Feisal's body.

The shaykh warned Abdel Rahman that sometimes it could be necessary to beat the jinn up: 'One of Feisal's jinn gave me the finger. Then he got beaten up. If he had spat on and hit the Quran he would really have been beaten up. This is how they should be treated. You force them to go out all the way to the little finger. Then you hold them there. When they have said the *shahāda* [testified to the truth of God], then you let them go.'

Some months after this conversation, I was contacted by one of Feisal's friends. He told me the shaykh in their mosque had suddenly refused to continue with the exorcisms. In contrast to his previous claims about Feisal being possessed by a rather alarming number of jinn, the shaykh now held the opinion that Feisal was suffering from a psychological disorder. Feisal's friend was not convinced by the shaykh. On behalf of Feisal he contacted me and asked if I could establish a contact with Abu Bilal, whom he knew I was working with. According to the friend, Feisal still had severe problems with jinn. I was happy to set up contact with Abu Bilal, but I made it clear to Abu Bilal that the previous shaykh had refused to read more *ruqya* for Feisal and that for some reason he had now identified Feisal's hardships as psychological in nature rather than jinn related. Abu Bilal agreed to meet Feisal and see to his problems.

We met in the mosque at 3 a.m. in March 2011. The plan was to first do the voluntary night prayer, *qiyām al-layl*. After the customary prayer, *raka'āt sunna*, performed when entering a mosque, I greet Feisal and ask how he is doing.

'*Al-ḥamdu li-l-Lāh* [praise to God],' he replies, 'it's hurting me – the knives, they cut me here in the legs.'

Abu Bilal starts the two-hour-long night prayer, followed by the obligatory prayer before daybreak, *ṣalāt al-fajr*. His recitation is much quieter than usual. Even the passionate supplications performed at the end of the prayer are carried out in a low voice.

After the prayers, we enter the small office of the mosque. Besides Feisal, Abu Bilal, and me, Erdam, a regular participant at the mosque, also comes along. Abu Bilal asks Feisal to sit in the black leather chair in the middle of the room. Abu Bilal then sits on a chair facing Feisal and takes his arm. He asks how Feisal is feeling: 'Are you afraid?'

Feisal confirms he is.

'How did you feel during the prayer?'

'I felt knives in my legs, they are cutting me.' Feisal's body starts to shake as he talks. He is much worse than I noticed in the mosque. Feisal does not speak Arabic and only very little Danish. He speaks Bosnian and some English. Abu Bilal speaks Danish and Arabic, but not English. I act as a translator between Abu Bilal and Feisal. Erdam speaks Turkish, Arabic, and Danish. He does not interfere in the conversation but sits ready behind Feisal's chair. Feisal says he is having trouble breathing. Abu Bilal asks if it is like this all the time.

'No, it just started now.'

Abu Bilal puts his right hand on Feisal's forehead and starts to recite the Quran close to Feisal's right ear. A few moments pass, then a muscle in Feisal's chest contracts, followed by a muscle on the other side of his chest. Then the whole of Feisal's upper body contracts. His eyelids are tightly closed. His shoulders move back and forth. The spasms intensify. Abu Bilal continues to recite and suddenly a pair of abnormal eyes stare out. Their focal point shifts in rapid jerks like the eyeballs of a bird.

I am sitting on the other side of a sofa table with my notepad and pen ready at hand. Then his eyes stare directly at me. I try not to be afraid. His mouth is wriggled into an odd grimace and the abrupt shakes in his body continue. Erdam holds Feisal's body from behind the black chair. Abu Bilal talks to the jinn in Arabic: 'Who are you? Get out from him.'

The jinn stammers indistinctly; the noises sound Arabic, but they are hard to decipher. The eyes move around madly, and then he starts to cry like a child.

'Are you Muslim?' Abu Bilal cries.

The jinn finally cries that its name is Amir. This is the first time we meet Amir. With his hand he makes the sign of the cross.

'You are a Christian.' Abu Bilal starts to recite again. The spasms reappear. Abu Bilal demands the jinn to say the *shahāda*: 'Say: "I witness that there is no god but God."' The jinn stutters, then changes the words, suddenly interrupted by making the sign of the cross. Abu Bilal recites again. The spasms intensify.

At last, the spirit complies and takes the Islamic creed. It is a relief for all of us. Apparently it disappears, but is then immediately replaced by a new spirit. It is not clear to me how the shift takes place, but now it is Muhammad, a Bosnian jinn, who has taken presence within Feisal's body.

'Do you speak Arabic?' cries Abu Bilal in Arabic. But the spirit does not speak Arabic. Abu Bilal tries instead with a few words in English: 'Go out, come out.'

The recitation continues for some time. At times the contractions seem to ease. Feisal sinks into the chair and blows through his mouth. He blows upwards so strongly that breath and spit hit Erdam, who wrenches his head away in disgust.

Abu Bilal tries to talk to the jinn again. The jinn answers. Now it grumbles in Arabic, but still refuses to obey the message of God. I am unsure whether this is still Muhammad, if the Arabic-speaking Amir has returned, or if yet another jinn has arrived. Abu Bilal gets angry. He moves close to Feisal's right ear and presses his right hand hard against his chest. He reads louder and faster, demands the Islamic creed, reads again. Nothing happens.

Abu Bilal walks out of the room. Erdam and I are left alone with Feisal and God knows how many jinn. The spasms continue but at a slower pace. He sits with his head looking down towards the floor. I walk to the other side of the table and sit down in front of him. I place my hands on his knees to make them relax. He looks at me – calm sad eyes – it is Feisal again.

'I can't control my body, *subḥān Allāh*.'

He speaks to me in English. He repeats the sentence on and on. '*Subḥān Allāh*, this is the will of God.'

## The agent and the patient

What happens inside Feisal when various jinn leave his body as others continue to arrive? How could this pain and apparent lack of control be the will of God? What should we understand by this statement? To find answers to these questions, let us consider some of the ways in which healing has been analysed in anthropology and in Danish psychiatry.

Building on John Dewey's claim that human experience is fundamentally characterised by uncertainty and ambiguity, Susan Whyte (1997) has described how people in Northern Uganda approach diviners, Catholic priests, biomedical doctors, and Muslim shaykhs not to get rid of uncertainty – which in any case would be impossible – but to establish a shelter of security against misfortune. As Whyte (1997: 3) points out, the precarity of life demands action. Going to the priest, the diviner, or the shaykh is one way for people to secure themselves against the arbitrary condition of human existence. In contrast to previous structuralist and functionalist studies of witchcraft and ritual that have tried to unpack the 'true' meanings of rituals, Whyte argues for an approach that sees ritual as a form of practical action, deployed by social agents in response to misfortune. According to Whyte, what is needed is a more naturalistic, lifelike, open-ended, and inconclusive anthropology that in the words of Rorty (1991a: 166) accepts 'our inheritance from, and our conversation with our fellow humans as our only source of guidance'. As Whyte (1997: 20) points out, a pragmatic ethnography requires above all 'that we see people as actors trying to alleviate suffering rather than as spectators applying cultural, ritual, or religious truths'.

Whyte's emphasis on the agency of people chimes with a wide range of medical anthropological studies that have aimed to destabilise all-encompassing structuralist models of healing in diverse ways (see e.g. Kleinman 1980, 1988; Mattingly 1998: 46). The same push towards recognising the agency and creative powers of humans, rather than seeing them merely as passive recipients, is expressed in Alyson Callan's (2012) study of mental health, modernity, and Islam in Bangladesh. In line with Whyte, Callan aims to destabilise the very concept of the 'patient'. Etymologically, 'patient' can be understood as a direct antonym of 'agent': that is, a passive recipient, 'a person who or thing which undergoes some action, or to which something is done' (OED 2019). Yet Callan shows how patients are not passive, but active agents in their own right.

According to Callan, the agency of patients is often severely constrained by power relations within their families, wider social structures, or the global economy that in a variety of ways dictate possible courses of action. Furthermore Callan's (2012: 201) interlocutors are frequently acted upon by invisible spirits, but although interfering spirits might momentarily displace consciousness, Callan found that the personal agency of the hosts is often increased. At times, encounters with spirits result in a heightened self-awareness through the mediation provided by healers. As Callan (2012: 199) concludes: 'Patients have agency. They visit healers who they know will give them the diagnosis they are seeking.'

In what sense can we understand Feisal, who was exorcised in the mosque, or Aziz, whom I followed during his psychiatric treatment, as patients and as agents? In Danish psychiatric healthcare the concept of the 'patient' has also been the object of critical debate (Gormsen 2006; Karlsson 2009; Barker and Buchanan-Barker 2009; Danish Council of Ethics 2012). Arguments parallel to Callan's have been made for a move towards more politically correct notions such as 'psychiatry user', 'citizen', or 'collaborator' (see e.g. Region Midtjylland 2009). 'User involvement' and 'free choice' have become key tropes of guidance in the management of psychiatric healthcare.

In an effort to establish a common set of values for the treatment of people with mental illnesses, the Ministries of the Interior, Health, and Social Affairs (2005: 11) have emphasised the importance of respect: 'Human beings with mental illnesses and their relatives are our collaborators. Their knowledge, insight, hope, resources, and attitude are crucial for the result of the procedures [*forløb*]. Respect is to recognise the individual human as unique with a right to self-determination of their own life and health.'

In addition these ministries emphasised the importance of meeting the psychiatric collaborators at eye level: 'Equality is a vital dimension of respectful interaction. It is our responsibility as professionals to ensure that the relation builds on equality and acknowledgement. As professionals we should accept the citizen as a unique and worthy person with a right to develop autonomously.'

In accordance with these reorientations of psychiatric treatment, but impatient with their slow implementation, proponents of the so-called 'recovery approach' have argued for a decidedly 'user-controlled psychiatry' (Jensen 2006; Klitgaard 2009). Under the banner of slogans such as 'You can do it. We can help', this approach aims to facilitate the development of social relationships, empowerment, social inclusion, and coping skills that may support a person's own potential for recovery. These efforts were widely appreciated and welcomed in the institutions where I did my fieldwork. Indeed, the Aarhus University Hospital in Risskov has been a leading partner in the development of a successful system for treating schizophrenia based on intensive, integrated, and multidisciplinary collaborations between social workers, nurses, psychiatrists, psychologists and, most importantly, the families of the mentally ill (OPUS 2007; see also Petersen et al. 2005; Thorup et al. 2005).

Yet most of the psychiatric personnel I met did not seem to depart fully from traditional psychiatric vocabulary in their daily work. Rather than 'psychiatry user', 'collaborator', or 'citizen', Aziz's psychiatrist Jørgen Aagaard preferred the more encompassing concept of a 'whole human' (*det hele menneske*, see Scene 6). However, in our conversations he would sometimes correct himself after using the word 'patient', adjusting his sentence to refer to 'the whole human'. I think these 'slips of the tongue' indicate that despite the impact of current user-oriented ideologies on Danish psychiatry, older notions such as the 'patient' still hold a continued importance (see also Luhrmann 2000: 128ff). Let us consider the possible sustained meanings or functions that the concept of the 'patient' and the modes of thinking it entails could have for both the psychiatric and the Islamic practices of healing I studied in Denmark.

What is it that happens when Feisal finally, in the jinn exorcism cited above, looks at me and says: 'I can't control my body, *subḥān Allāh*, this is the will of God.' We could, in line with Whyte and Callan, read this as the utterance of a patient who aimed at and succeeded in finding a healer who could provoke the symptoms of the diagnosis he hoped to obtain. Yet we need to be cautious here. First of all, it was not Feisal but his friend who found the healer, using me as an intermediary. In many of the possession cases I know of, the patients are initially reluctant to accept treatment – a reluctance which often is interpreted as the effect of the devil's whispering. To read Feisal's statement as the fulfilment of his own desire for a specific diagnosis would also be in direct contradiction with his own understanding of the situation.

A more immediate interpretation would be to see his utterance simply as a realisation and acknowledgement that occurred as a result of the treatment. My hunch is that this utterance might be applied quite literally as a definition of what it means to become a patient in the original sense of the word. That is, persons who are able to endure actions inflicted upon them by others.

Within the Islamic framework, patience (*ṣabr*), along with trust (*tawakkul*) and thankfulness (*shukr*), are the most important virtues that may be cultivated when an ill person (*marīḍ*) suffers the hardships of an illness. Abu Bilal would exemplify this with the story of Job, who not only endured the loss of his children, his wife, his friends, and his wealth, but whose physical body was reduced by painful and prolonged illnesses to mere skin and bones. Yet in all these misfortunes, Job remained steadfast in his gratitude to God. As stated in Surat Sad: 'Indeed, We found him patient, an excellent servant. Indeed, he was one repeatedly turning back [to God]' (Quran 38: 44).

To be sure, this emphasis on patience and the patient as a person being acted upon stands in conflict with the dominant notions of agency in medical anthropology, as well as the current 'consumer' or 'user' oriented discourses within Danish psychiatry. Yet I think it is of key importance to understanding what healing entails, both in psychiatric settings and in Islamic traditions of exorcism. The main question here is not whether or to what degree patients have agency, and nor is it about how a system of healing could be organised so as to 'respect' rather than deprive patients of their agency. Of course patients have agency, sometimes even too much of it, but both psychiatric healthcare and Islamic exorcisms seem mainly to be about redirecting the agency of patients and disrupting their capacity to destroy themselves.

As pointed out by Mahmood (2005: 8), the understanding of agency in academic debates is often framed within the idiom of resistance: 'the capacity to realize one's own interests against the weight of custom, tradition, transcendental will, or other obstacles.' In making this claim, Mahmood addresses a number of feminist studies that like Whyte and Callan have aimed to locate a space for female agency in the Muslim world (see e.g. Abu-Lughod 1986; Altorki 1986; Wikan 1991). Discussing Boddy's (1989) work on the *zār* cult in Northern Sudan, Mahmood points out how here too, female spirit mediums come to stand in for such an autonomous consciousness, articulated against the hegemonic male cultural norms of

Muslim societies. As Boddy (1989: 345) writes, to take spirit possession seriously as a medium for the cultivation of women's consciousness requires a 'consideration of women as actors in their world'. Yet, as Mahmood makes clear, there are modes of self-realisation where action and agency are not dependent on the ability of an individual to assert their will against the presence of norms or other external forces.

Drawing on Foucault's (1997) analysis of ethical formation, Mahmood claims that self-realisation may indeed also be located in the ability of a subject to align and cultivate itself in accordance with external forces and authorities. Mahmood applies this notion of 'ethical formation' in order to account for the agency of pious Egyptian women whose self-realisation is dependent not on their ability to enforce their will against the 'oppressive' norms of their society, but on their success in fashioning themselves by actively embodying the virtues of the Prophet Muhammad. Here we may note the parallels with the idea of 'non-resisting' freedom in the work of Merleau-Ponty (2002: 529) and Lévi-Strauss (1983: 12, see Chapter 1). To explain this peculiar compliant modality of agency, Mahmood provides the example of a virtuoso musician who submits herself to painful disciplinary practice and hierarchical apprenticeship in order to acquire the ability to play her instrument. As Mahmood (2005: 29) observes:

> Importantly, her agency is predicated upon her ability to be taught, a condition classically referred to as 'docility'. Although we have come to associate docility with the abandonment of agency, the term literally implies the malleability required of someone in order for her to be instructed in a particular skill or knowledge – a meaning that carries less a sense of passivity than one of struggle, effort, exertion, and achievement.

In a similar analytical move, Asad (2003) has described the agency that may reside in inhabiting the space of pain. To associate pain with agency may seem grotesque, since pain in our modern secular age is often identified as that which all our capacities for action should aim to minimise. Is pain not something which happens when personal agency has become dysfunctional? Surely to be in pain is to be ruled by forces that, if one had sufficient power, one would seek to eliminate. Yet Asad claims that there are forms of suffering that cannot simply be reduced to a passive experience. In that very situation in which all attempts at action in the external world have been disabled due to severe pain, there may still be the possibility of inhabiting pain, allowing its work on the body, and cultivating the way in which pain is lived (see also Kleinman 2012: 609; Pandolfo 2018: 330).

When Feisal expresses that his condition is the will of God, I think we should understand it exactly in this way – that is, as an expression and cultivation of the virtue of patience in confrontation with pain. With reference to examples ranging from early Christian martyrs to birthing mothers and Oedipus, Asad (2003: 69) points out that pain in this sense 'is not simply a *cause* of action, but can also itself be a *kind* of action' (emphasis in the original). Both Asad and Mahmood point to forms of agency that may be located not in the ability to act outwardly, but in the ways one can let oneself be taught or endure the actions of an outside force. We could thus make a distinction between, on the one hand, agency as the capacity to act and exert power; and, on the other hand, agency as the process of receiving, allowing, inhabiting, or even acting out the actions of something else: that is, being an agent.[2] To be sure, this latter notion of agency comes close to the classical definition of the patient. What are the procedures by which healers may foster the virtues that enable patients to let themselves be acted upon?

## Iconoclasm

Much of the material I present here could be framed, in line with Whyte's analysis, as pragmatic reactions to the precarity and misfortunes of life. Often patients express great distress and uncertainty over their precarious situation, but in the actual healing encounters their problems appear not to be framed around the issue of uncertainty. Rather, a key problem addressed by psychiatrists, nurses, and shaykhs is that of already established certainties. That a patient has approached a healer indicates that already, at this early stage, a degree of self-diagnosis has been made and a course of action planned. Indeed, this is the agency of which Callan speaks (2012; see also Zola 1973). Common to both psychiatric treatment and Islamic exorcisms is, however, the great emphasis on the necessity of external healing agencies – namely God or biomedicine.

In both psychiatry and Islam, these externalities are understood as lying beyond the power of ordinary humans. In the healing encounter, it becomes the task of the healer to prepare the patient in such a way that these external agencies may be allowed to do their work: that is, to help them become patients. This involves building up a number of hindrances, or what Emilie Gomart (2002) in a different context has termed 'generous constraints', that allow the patients to escape from any illusions of being able to correctly perceive and autonomously act against the forces causing their suffering. The problem here is often not uncertainty or existential angst, but rather the certainties, half certainties, and already-taken-for-granted understandings of one's own suffering. For this reason the task of the healer becomes that of disrupting the certainties of patients, so as to produce a situation where patients realise that protection and healing are ultimately beyond their own capacity. In other words, the initial task of the healer is not to provide a response to uncertainty, but to produce uncertainty. It is from this ground of deep existential doubt – the realisation that one's knowledge and capacity for perception is deficient – that the healer may then invite the patient to take the leap and allow themselves to be healed from the outside.

This oscillation between doubt and certitude is a critical requirement for the healing practices of psychiatrists, nurses, and Muslim shaykhs. I have come to understand this oscillation as related to a kind of 'image-production' and iconoclastic 'image-destruction'. I use the word image in the broadest possible definition to denote what Latour (2002: 16) in his essay on iconoclasm calls 'any sign, work of art, inscription, or picture that acts as a mediation to access something else'. This oscillation between efforts to render visible on the one hand and the sabotage or defacement of visibility on the other is inherent in many traditions of mystical revelation (see e.g. Pandolfo 1997; Taussig 1999; Steinbock 2007). Here I relate it to what one of Kierkegaard's (2005) many personas, Johannes de Silentio, identified as the two 'movements of infinity' that are involved in the particular state of mind he calls faith.

In the first movement I locate the doubts and uncertainties of both patients and healers. This, in the words of De Silentio (Kierkegaard 2005: 51), is the movement of resignation. It is the realisation of the arbitrary and unjust character of human life, the recognition that all the images and knowledge one had of the world are embarrassingly deficient and flooded with error. This is the movement that takes place in the realisation that indeed any true vision in this world is impossible. The second movement takes place when both healer and patient, having first renounced the finite, visible world, take it up again in full knowledge of the impossibility of doing so. To be sure, this is an absurd movement and, as Kierkegaard's De Silentio (2005[1843]: 55) makes clear, it can only occur through the suspension of one's disbelief in the finite and visible world through a leap of faith.

Here I identify these movements of faith not only in the ongoing oscillation between visibility and invisibility that may be working within the healer and the patient, but also in the fluctuating positions taken up in the healing interaction between patient and healer. Indeed I suggest that the healers themselves need to become 'patients' before they can take the leap of faith required in the act of healing. Certainly there are vast differences between psychiatric treatments and Islamic exorcisms, but for me the greater surprise has been that despite clear and visible differences, structural similarities do appear to exist. When asked to reflect on one another's practices, Muslim shaykhs and psychiatric practitioners alike tend to emphasise their differences, identifying the other as remnants of a bygone past or as agents of a morally corrupt system of oppression. Yet healers in both traditions frame their criticisms and diagnoses in strikingly similar ways. In so doing, they engage in what, with Latour (2002), I will describe as 'image-making' and 'image-breaking'.

Sometimes, however, the breaking of the images of the other is also the breaking of one's own. To properly understand this oscillation between existential doubt and faith, between the invisibility and visibility involved in becoming a patient, requires us to take a close look at how healers themselves perceive and analyse their own and one another's practices.

## Angels cannot enter a room with images on the wall

The psychiatrist Jørgen, the psychiatric nurse Esther, and I are watching the video of Nadia, the young Bosnian woman being diagnosed for infestations of jinn through Quranic recitation (see Scene 5 and Scene 6).

Abu Bilal has read verses from the Quran over a jar of water, which the woman has to drink. In addition he has purified the house, in particular her and her sister's bedroom. He has asked her to take down all the family photos and posters of Marilyn Monroe and *Sex in the City* that lined the walls. Such photos and posters – containing what Abu Bilal refers to as 'soul', that is, depicting human beings or animals – make it impossible for angels to enter the room. If angels cannot enter the room, *shayṭān* and evil jinn can do whatever they want. Abu Bilal tells the woman that this might very well be the reason why she and her sister have been having such terrible nightmares.

During his reading in the room, he has also discovered a strange-looking image containing a form of writing that appeared to mimic Quranic text but which definitely was not. The woman's father explained that the text was meant to protect against the evil eye – the harmful destructive gaze that may be induced by people's conscious or unconscious envy. Abu Bilal makes it clear that the image on her wall does not protect her at all, and that in fact it has the opposite effect. Since the scriptures on the image are not of Quranic origin, only appearing to look like it, they are evidently magic – *siḥr.*

Magic essentially operates by polluting and subverting the divine message. Abu Bilal would often explain how the magician (*sāḥir*) takes a piece of hair, some blood, nails, or other impure substances and puts them together with verses of the Quran. Sometimes the magician will write Quranic verses backwards, or change their meaning. At times the *sāḥir* will even write obscene things in menstrual blood or semen. What happens then is that evil jinn are attracted to it, and as a favour to the magician – who by his evil acts has stepped over to their side (the side of the eternally condemned, *al-rajīm*) – they will let him make use of their powers. The jinn will pretend to have become his slaves. The magician may be able to assume superhuman powers and direct invisible harm to his victims, but often, however, he will be unaware that it is the evil jinn who have taken possession of him.

While the photos and posters on the walls need only be hidden inside the drawers, Abu Bilal advises Nadia and her father to destroy the piece of magic they had framed and hung above the bed for protection:

'This only makes it worse. It's strictly forbidden by God (*ḥarām*). Against envy you say "I seek refuge in God, Lord of the daybreak" and "I seek refuge in God, Lord of humankind". These verses are from the Quran. When you read them, envy can never harm you. If you read Surat al-Falaq and al-Nas every day – when I have read it here – it's impossible for envy to enter. This one [the image] is like magic. I swear by God. Look. There is nothing of the Quran. It's like cards and magic. It's magic and this is a picture of the imam.[3] Impossible, it's forbidden, do you understand? It will never protect you from envy. God protects. Quran protects. Not this one. Perhaps this is a bigger problem – more dangerous than the images. So I don't think you should have it here. Just destroy it and throw it out. This is not Quran. Don't doubt, 100 per cent, believe me. I swear by God that it creates more damage.'

Jørgen, Esther, and I watch the video. This is one of the clearest examples I have of the form of iconoclasm that is at work in the Islamic tradition of healing. It is not, however, iconoclasm as classified by Latour (2002: 27) as 'the total war against all images'. Rather, it is iconoclasm against 'freeze-framing'. The problem neo-orthodox Muslims have with images is not the existence of images as such. As described in the previous chapter, neo-orthodox Muslims use visual imagery for a wide variety of purposes. Moving images such as the film we recorded are not a problem at all, nor are photographic images problematic as long as they are kept in a drawer and only occasionally brought out for display. But if images containing what Abu Bilal refers to as 'soul' hang freely on a wall, as if the soul in them was eternally watching over the room, then they risk losing the sense of impermanence inherent to all earthly life and open the possibility of heretic veneration (*shirk*).[4] Indeed they risk becoming abodes for jinn. Combining a drawing of a mortal shaykh with fake imitations of Quranic verses and hanging this above the bed as a protection against the evil eye is even worse. The distorted replica of the incomparable, eternal, and divine words should be immediately removed and destroyed.

As we watch the video of Abu Bilal, Nadia, and her father, I observe both senior health professionals crease their eyebrows. I try to imagine what it is they see. Just a moment ago, Jørgen and Esther watched another piece of footage in which a shaykh tapped a small amount of blood from the back of a patient through the technique widely known as cupping (*ḥijāma*, al-Jawziyah 2003[1292–1350 C.E.]: 59ff). Blood from the outer layer of the skin of the back is believed to collect waste. Partly because evil jinn prefer to live in filthy places, my interlocutors argue that it became a prophetic practice to remove a bit of blood as a method of prevention and protection against possession. Clearly not agreeing with this explanation, Jørgen told me about the great significance of placebo in all healthcare. His explanation was strongly critical and, to use Michael Taussig's (1999: 3) vocabulary, even defacing of the truth-value of this peculiar practice of healing through blood tapping. Yet in a curious way Jørgen's defacement of the Islamic healing practices also evolved into a self-critique, a kind of self-defacement:

'We're allowed to reveal that it is the procedures in contact with a human being that count the most.' Jørgen continues: 'We can give a pedagogical example. In the case of Rheumatoid Arthritis [*leddegigt*] you use gold [or] salazopyrin – right.'

Esther laughs knowingly.

'First you bind a band around here [the arm] and then the gold is injected. For 60 per cent this reduces Rheumatoid Arthritis within 14 days – those swelling joints. If instead you inject salt water – if you use placebo – and everything looks exactly the same – you lift it up, shake it, attend to it [*ordner det*] … then if before, 60 per cent had the swelling of their joints reduced, then now it is perhaps 45 per cent. This is because the more procedures that are tied to the healing agent, the greater the placebo effect, right? It is not enough with words. Preferably something more needs to be added. When something is added, then placebo is strengthened … In all treatments, there is a massive psychological element in addition to the biomedical.'

'Which results in self-healing,' Esther adds.

'Which results in self-healing – and at rather high percentages,' Jørgen repeats. Esther nods approvingly.

Jørgen continues: 'In the case of depression, it's often difficult, this I can also give as an example. If you treat 100 patients once a week, and they're being rated with the Hamilton Rating Scale … and they talk with a nice nurse or psychiatrist for half an hour for 6–12 weeks, and one group gets tablets of chalk and the other gets medicine, then we need a very, very large number of patients – 200, 300, maybe 400 – before a difference can be seen between treatment with medicine and treatment with placebo. But if you had just given the medicine and said, *eat* and come back in 14 days or 3 weeks – if you did not have that weekly control of symptoms – then it won't help … The basic principle is that the more special and developed the placebo is, the better it works.'

The discussion continues for a while. I ask if it is this small but significant difference between treatment with medicine and placebo that justifies treatment with medicine despite all the reported side effects. Jørgen replies that in fact it is rather the difference between merely prescribing medicine as compared to meeting and talking to the patient once a week. What he means by this is that meeting the patient once a week is simply regarded as being too expensive, even though it would evidently be more effective.

'In this area the Church is competitive,' he adds.

We have viewed Abu Bilal's purification of the house, the removal of images in Nadia's bedroom, and the identification of magic hanging above her bed, supposedly to protect against envy. Jørgen makes it clear to me that what we are watching here is in fact an instance of a universal psychological phenomenon, namely the battle between good and evil. He sees, however, a major difference between this distinction, as conceived in modern psychiatry as an internal dichotomy doing its work within all human beings, and what he identifies in my video as reminiscent of practices predating the Protestant Reformation in Europe, where evil was to be located as an external agent outside the body of man. I do not agree with Jørgen that we can so sharply distinguish between a definition of evil as either external to or internal and ever-present in man. In fact I don't think he completely agrees with it himself, but I see why he makes such a judgement from the images he was presented with. If my footage feeds into these dichotomies, this is a problem I need to do something about.

Then Jørgen and Esther add an important observation:

'It's very authoritarian. The priests [shaykhs] are very authoritative. They are absolutely certain in what they do. This is another cultural way of looking at it,' says Jørgen.

Esther continues: 'It sounded as if it was his decision, "This needs to be removed and this needs to be removed." Could another shaykh have said, "This one has to be removed, but this one can stay on the wall"?'

I reply: 'There are a lot of variations on this. Some would say that images are allowed to stay on the wall here. There are differing opinions about it. You refer to differing descriptions of the practices of the Prophet and there can be discussions about how to interpret the texts. This is why there are different practices.'

Esther interrupts: 'But then they get a lot of personal impact, I mean, their impact becomes very dependent on the person.'

I agree, 'Yes.'

Jørgen nods approvingly: 'Very authoritarian.'

Esther to Jørgen: 'You could say that in our system we are more dependent on context. We keep statistics and create lists, who responds and who does not, what is being shown.'

Jørgen laughs: 'You mean in psychiatry?'

Throughout the conversation he is hesitant about Esther's and my comparison between psychiatry and Islamic healing. Rather, he sees the relevant comparison as between Islamic forms of healing and medieval Christian practices and understandings of healing.

In this case, however, Jørgen agrees with Esther's comparison, and then again emphasises that, indeed, 'It's very authoritarian. Paternalistic, we might call it. Very, very authoritarian. *It is like this*.'

Esther adds: 'It's not so evidence based.'

Jørgen: 'There's no doubt in his mind, I think this is very interesting, because it unveils a very authoritarian – in his case, right – it makes the religion very authoritative. It is like this, right. I think this is a bit interesting.'

## Placebo

Let us consider more closely what happens when the practitioners of the dominant system of healing in Denmark are allowed to dissect and deface the healing practices of a minority group. The result is perhaps predictable. Two key themes are compared, highlighted, and ranked: the locus of evil, and the right to authority. Jørgen and Esther point out how evil in Islamic healing is located as a force external to the patient. In contrast, the Western psychiatric model recognises that both good and evil are an inherent existential fact internal to all human life. And while the Islamic healer, in Jørgen and Esther's view, seems to obtain authority from within his own person, Western psychiatry has scientific procedures for developing and verifying forms of healing that go beyond the impact of particular human agencies. In summary, Jørgen concludes that the alternative healing practices of Islam, while they may exist in our contemporary world, are in fact better located in an evolutionary epoch quite distant from our own, namely the Middle Ages.

As Johannes Fabian (2002) points out, it is a widely used classificatory strategy to identify 'the time of the other' as a remnant of a bygone past in this way. Identifying the Middle Ages as the time proper to Islamic practice is a common theme in secular Danish discourse (see e.g. Hervik 2004, 2006; see also Said 1995). But Jørgen and Esther's message is more complex than this. Having only these brief visual recordings at their disposal, they are forced to attribute to them the knowledge they have of healing from their own practices – thereby rendering the 'other', as Levinas (see Wyschogrod 2002: 191) would have it, into the 'same'. A process of mirroring – or what in the language of psychoanalysis could be called 'transference' (Freud 1959[1912]) – starts when Jørgen compares the injection of gold in the treatment of Rheumatoid Arthritis with the removal of impure blood or the intake of purified water in the Islamic treatment. In a peculiar way, their description of Islamic healing practices becomes a reflection on aspects of their own healing practices.

Jørgen argues there is an essential difference between locating evil as something internal to the patient in modern psychiatry, and the externalisation and expulsion of evil at work in Islamic healing practices. However, in many other contexts psychiatrists would argue against the internalisation of evil that has characterised past psychiatric models of the human interior. In fact much work is currently being done to liberate patients from identifications with illness that assume their entire being, such as: 'I am a schizophrenic, depressed, or bipolar.'

Esther once made the importance of this clear to me by drawing a parallel with physical illnesses. As she said: 'You might *have* influenza, but you *are not* influenza. The same should apply to mental illnesses.' Hence modern psychiatry works towards an objectification of psychiatric illnesses such that they may be conceived as separate, or at least do not entirely coincide with the being of the patient.[5] Indeed the shift in terminology from 'patient' towards 'psychiatry user' indicates, among other things, the way in which the institution aims to distance itself from a model in which psychiatric illness consumes the full identity of the suffering person. The modern 'psychiatry user' may suffer from schizophrenia, but 'schizophrenic patients' as such should not exist.

Jørgen has also been an advocate for a much less rigid use of psychiatric diagnoses. In other contexts he promotes a treatment of schizophrenia and psychosis that indeed takes seriously the voices people may be hearing. In the book *Controlling the Voices* (Nielsen, Mikkelsen, and Aagaard 2009), Jørgen and his colleagues propose a system for mastering voices based on the insight that two-thirds of people who hear voices in fact never contact the psychiatric system (see also Romme and Escher 2000; International Community for Hearing Voices 2012). Hence hearing voices cannot in and of itself be regarded as pathological. Rather, it is the way in which one hears them and the manner in which they act on the voice-hearer that may develop into a condition that requires psychiatric intervention. For these reasons Jørgen and his colleagues advocate that treatment should not be about 'downplaying or exterminating the voices, but about listening to their message' (Nielsen, Mikkelsen, and Aagaard 2009: 7; see also Luhrmann 2012a).

As Romme and Escher (2000) describe in a study of 'non-patients' with voice-hearing, this peculiar phenomenon often seems to be caused either by an irresolvable life situation or trauma, a conflict between ideals and reality, or obstacles to the voice-hearer's personal development. Voices can also emerge as a defence against overwhelming emotions that cannot be contained within consciousness. Finally, voices can be carriers of metaphorical meaning, bearing witness and giving voice to experiences of repression or harm that a person may unconsciously have suppressed. As Nielsen, Mikkelsen, and Aagaard (2009: 8) state, 'voices can be a symptom of an unresolved problem'. Indeed the voices function as 'messengers with information about the problem', and they will continue to be present for as long as the problem exists.

This form of therapy, aiming to listen to and in some way take seriously the messages of voices, is reminiscent of a wide range of traditional spirit possession cures described in the ethnographic literature around the world (see e.g. Crapanzano and Garrison 1977; Crapanzano 1985; Connor, Asch, and Asch 1986; Turner 1989; Boddy 1989, 1994; Maarouf 2007; Drieskens 2008). In her work on the Islamic treatment of *ruqya shar'iyya* in Morocco, Pandolfo (2011: 32; 2018: 265ff) explores how unresolved traumas and experiences of loss that evolve into the mute, inaccessible state of melancholia can be addressed through the manifestation of the jinn (see also Freud 2001[1917]). According to Pandolfo, the Quranic recitation works to reveal the unjust tyranny of the jinn, but it may also disclose and bear witness to the madness, hypocrisy, and injustices of the social world in which the patient is embedded. However, in contrast to the Islamic case – with its emphasis on the submission of the patient, jinn, and healer to an all-powerful God – the solution for voice-hearing for Jørgen and his colleagues is to learn how to control them. As they state, 'one needs to become master of them … dialogue with voices has the best effect as long as there is no doubt that it is the voice hearer who is "the boss"' (Nielsen, Mikkelsen, and Aagaard 2009: 8).

In this method of treatment a similar form of autonomy is ascribed to the voice-hearer as is proposed in the arguments for a clearer separation of the psychiatry user from psychiatric illnesses. To take such voices seriously entails seeing them as something separable from the kernel of the individual, as a form of external agency with which one can reason and even make certain arrangements regarding when and where they should appear so that one is not constantly disturbed (Nielsen, Mikkelsen, and Aagaard 2009: 61). However, as we sit watching the videos from my fieldwork in the mosques, Jørgen sees no parallels between his own and these Islamic treatments. Instead Jørgen seems to present a somewhat conservative stance, despite the fact that much recent psychiatry is now trying to incorporate elements from 'pre-modern' healing practices that seek precisely to convolute and externalise evil so that it does not pollute the entirety of the suffering soul.

## Authority

Later in my discussion with Jørgen and Esther we return to the central question of authority. I ask if some form of authoritarian intervention is not also central to the interaction between patient and healer in psychiatric healthcare: if the psychiatrist and the nurse must not also take on a measure of authority at the moment of healing. Jørgen and Esther completely agree. To be sure, this is also implicit in the discussion about placebo. Injecting salt water or handing out tablets of chalk without authorising it with medical procedures simply does not help anything, as Jørgen asserts and as has been widely recognised in studies of placebo (see e.g. Harrington 2000a; Kirsch 2000).

The issue of authority comes up again when we have viewed the sequence of the meeting between Jørgen and his patient Aziz, who was committed to treatment after being diagnosed with paranoid schizophrenia (Scene 4). At first, Jørgen listened attentively to and acknowledged the story of how Aziz became a victim of his second wife's magic, was possessed by an evil jinn, and then was finally healed through recitation of the Quran (see Chapter 2). After acknowledging Aziz's own account of his illness, Jørgen then brought forth the indisputable fact that Aziz had to comply with: 'It's not only the imam who has done a good job. It's also because of the medicine … The medicine helps you to control your own thoughts.'

This statement is clearly in direct contradiction with Aziz's own understanding of the situation. What Aziz tries to assert here, as on several other occasions, is that he is already cured of his illness. The cure, in Aziz's understanding, was Islam. The continued psychiatric medication is not simply redundant. In Aziz's view, it is harming him by exhausting his consciousness, thereby making it difficult for him to fulfil his religious obligations. This is difficult for Aziz to state in the present situation because he knows the psychiatrist and nurse will conceive of his self-analysis as a symptom of an upcoming psychosis. As Esther once said: 'When Aziz becomes psychotic, he becomes religious.'

Jørgen knows well the thoughts Aziz has about his forced medication. Yet here he chooses to directly ignore and overrule them by stating the positive effects of medication as a fact beyond dispute. For Aziz there is no way out of the conversation other than to somehow comply with Jørgen's statement: 'It helps me to sleep,' Aziz declares. While sleeping has in fact been difficult for Aziz due to severe nightmares, his statement about the effects of the medicine on sleep is ambiguous. While apparently serving to fulfil Jørgen's demand for compliance, it also carries a tacit critique, since sleepiness and generally being exhausted and drugged is exactly what makes it difficult for Aziz to practise the religious duties he sees as central to his cure. As the jinn who once possessed Aziz tried to escape from testifying to the 'truth of God' during the exorcisms, another part of Aziz is now trying to escape giving in to the demands of the psychiatrist for testifying to the 'truth of psychotropic medicine'.

When Aziz, his wife, and I watched a preliminary version of the film in autumn 2012, he started to laugh. It was evident how both he and Jørgen were deliberately misunderstanding one another's statements in this situation. The incongruity of seeing himself explain how the medication exhausts him and makes him tired apparently called for some form of release. Aziz's wife added that the problem was no longer that he could not sleep, but rather that he slept all the time.

While being fully aware of this resistance within Aziz, Jørgen and Esther continued to assert the beneficial effects of medicine in all their meetings with him. The strategy they used was not so much to outreason Aziz, which would entail a critique of his story of the magic and the jinn; indeed they actively acknowledged Aziz's own account. Simultaneously, however, they asked him to verbally repeat in his own words the contradictory account about the beneficial effects of medicine, as if verbal repetition of these effects would eventually force Aziz to give in and comply with the medical treatment he had been sentenced to take. This pedagogical method of shaping a consciousness through continued verbal repetition bears a similarity to the cultivation of ethical sensitivities in the recitation and memorisation of the Quran in the mosques (see Hirschkind 2006: 80). The similarity is perhaps most clearly illustrated in Scene 8 where Aziz becomes subject to quite a thorough biomedical reprogramming from his nurse, Esther (see Chapter 6 for further discussion of this scene).

In all this, a contradiction seems to be taking shape. We may recall how Aziz's nurse Esther emphasised the notion of 'self-healing' in our discussion with Jørgen about placebo. Indeed both Esther and Jørgen seem to be saying that the greatest evidential effects of psychiatric medicine in fact derive from placebo. In framing placebo as an effect of 'self-healing', Esther seems to be moving towards the analytical framework of medical anthropologists such as Whyte and Callan, who argue for an understanding of healing as generated through forms of agency that originate essentially in the socially human. Here Esther appears to hold the widely accepted conviction that a given medication can only heal insofar as the patient believes in it (see also Kirsch 2000; Johansen and Hvidt 2003). Yet in her interaction with Aziz, Esther takes on a considerably more determinate position. Now she appears to be saying that these drugs work regardless of what you believe. Hence her job is to make Aziz understand their effects, in order to ensure he will actually take them.

Quite a considerable amount of certainty is displayed when Esther and Jørgen correct Aziz's statement that the antipsychotic drug Zyprexa only helps him to sleep by stating how in fact it also works to make him psychologically stronger. Week after week, Aziz is repeatedly made to testify to these indisputable facts. The repeated recitation of the beneficial effects of antipsychotic medication lies close to that of religious testimony. Aziz, however, is a complex entity in this battle. A part within him seems to comply and accept the beneficial effects of biomedicine, while another part seems to resist by somewhat sarcastically testifying to 'sleepiness' as the essential outcome of antipsychotics. It is this resistant part within Aziz that, in the optics of Jørgen and Esther, is closely related to religious delusion and perhaps even an upcoming psychosis. It is this that has to be overpowered in order to ensure that Aziz starts taking the medicine, so that it may be allowed to do its work on his body.[6]

## Psychological problems

When I asked the shaykhs in the mosques about the treatments offered by Danish psychiatry, they were usually quite explicit in their critique. Some of my interlocutors would even claim that practising and truly faithful Muslims are unable to have psychological problems. As pointed out by Abu Samir (see also Chapter 1), Danish psychiatry was often identified as an instrument of evil. As he asserted: 'The problem is that the Danish system drags people down. They want us to be like them, but we cannot.'

Discussing the time when he himself was taking antidepressants, Abu Samir concluded that: 'If you use these things you lose. [People] don't know that they lose, but step by step the drugs start to control their lives.' In Abu Samir's view illness is not treated but rather produced by psychiatric healthcare. To 'lose' and become infected with the illnesses of Danish psychiatry means to be deprived of the ability to hear and obey the divine message. According to Abu Samir, a proper ethical life is thereby made impossible. Abu Samir's critique of the modern institution runs parallel to those reported by Pandolfo's (2007: 335, 348) Moroccan interlocutors when describing the increasing spread of despair (*qanaṭ*) among young Moroccans – a condition that leads to the loss of all hope and to the temptation of doing away with life – a state of mad living death (*ḥumq*) with no possibility of return. As we shall see in the next chapter, Abu Samir's critique of the psychiatric system also shows a symmetry with Jørgen's view as he points out how Islamic exorcisms can be dangerous to psychologically vulnerable people.

For Abu Samir, however, the danger of being exposed to the Danish system compelled him to return to his country of origin together with his Danish wife and their two children. As a political refugee, Abu Samir knew he risked being imprisoned upon his return, but he calculated that imprisonment was a lesser threat than the risk involved in prolonged exposure to the Danish system and what he regarded as the degenerate, numb Muslim population in Denmark.

While Abu Samir's analysis of Danish psychiatry may seem extreme, it was shared by many Muslims in the communities where I worked.

However, some shaykhs would be less definitive in their critique and would find exceptions where treatment with psychiatric medicine was in fact necessary. Thus in Abu Bilal's view, some patients are so ill it is virtually impossible to call them back to life. For him, medication is necessary if a patient becomes suicidal or dangerous to others. To drive its victim to commit suicide is, according to Abu Bilal, the ultimate victory for a malevolent jinn. But in his view, the majority of psychiatric cases would be better treated and prevented by regular attendance at the mosque (see e.g. Scene 9).

As also pointed out by Abu Samir and Aziz, the problem with psychiatric medication is that it makes proper Islamic practice, such as keeping prayer times and allowing the heart to be touched by Quranic recitations, difficult. With a few exceptions, Abu Bilal agreed with Abu Samir and Aziz that the treatment offered by Danish psychiatric healthcare can be harmful. This is not, however, because doctors are intentionally evil. Rather, it is because the doctors themselves are ill – consumed by the earthly visible world (*dunyā*) and ignorant of God's guidance (in *jāhiliyya*). In this critique a certain temporality is also implied. Thus while Jørgen identified the proper time of Islamic healing practices as the Middle Ages, Abu Bilal argued that psychiatrists and psychiatric patients were often led astray by the scientific certainties of the modern epoch – a moment in time where people are increasingly alienated and consumed by worldly matters.

In contrast with these views, Abu Abdallah, a shaykh from a neighbouring town, explained that he saw it as his primary job to redirect people who thought they had been possessed by jinn to proper treatment in psychiatric healthcare. This shaykh held a degree in psychology. According to Abu Abdallah, only one out of a hundred patients he received had truly been afflicted by jinn. His work consisted in reading a few verses of the Quran to the patient. When nothing seemed to happen, the patient would have to proceed to psychiatric treatment.

The shaykh's renunciation of the effectiveness of *ruqya* for treating most of his patients continues to puzzle me. It parallels the views of several other Muslims who have gone through higher education and who frequently deny that creatures such as jinn could ever enter the world of humans. It is in some ways a more radical position than that of Abu Samir or Abu Bilal, for what this shaykh in fact claims is that two different ontologies of illness are operating at the same time.[7] Possession by jinn and a psychiatric diagnosis such as psychosis are for this shaykh not just different ways of talking about the same phenomena, as I am sometimes inclined to think; they are, in his view, entirely different phenomena. While this shaykh severely downplays the effectiveness and relevance of his own healing practices, he was praised by several of my interlocutors as one of the best healers in Scandinavia.

## Breaking and making

At first glance the dissimilarities between Islamic exorcisms and psychiatric treatments appear as striking. While one treatment primarily emphasises the intake of psychiatric drugs, the other works through procedures of loud Quranic recitation and intense corporeal contact. While psychiatric encounters usually take place in the manner of a conversation, with participants sitting around a table in a somewhat impersonalised institutional setting, the Islamic exorcisms are embedded in familiar surroundings, with the participants grouped closely together on the carpet in the patient's home or in the mosque. Nevertheless, the ways in which Muslim healers move between statements about jinn possession and diagnoses of psychiatric disorders, certainty and uncertainty, show a significant resemblance to the movements of the nurses and psychiatrists between renunciations and affirmations of psychiatric treatments.

Both the psychiatric and Islamic healers I worked with were keen to make the differences between their systems of treatment clear to me. Yet it is not only the way in which the proponents of the two healing systems talk about and attempt to denounce each other's practices that are similar. The basic structure of taking on authority as a healer, designating beyond doubt, and carrying out healing practices also shares a common ground. The certitude Abu Bilal ascribes to his patients is exemplified by his own actions in the act of healing. So is it with Jørgen, who, without a shred of doubt, attempts to enforce upon Aziz that psychiatric medicine is not poison but healing.

At this moment of certitude they are like Hastrup (1992) as she explains the real meaning of the secret invisible ritual being performed behind the visible facades of the Icelandic ram exhibition, or the shaykh in the YouTube video as he exposes a '7000 year old jinn inside man' as undeniable visual evidence of the existence of this invisible category of malevolent spirits (see Chapter 3). The certitude displayed in the act of healing seems, however, to stand in marked contrast to the renunciation of any true capacity to heal that psychiatrists, nurses, shaykhs, and patients also frequently express.

As Latour (2002) makes clear, the perceived danger and problem so many people have with visual images is that they too easily become reified as something in and of themselves (see also Keane 2013). Against the compulsion of smashing the idols of others, as exemplified by both Islamic and Christian forms of iconoclasm but arguably also in the academic discipline of deconstructivist criticism, Latour (2002: 25; 2004) ironically points out that it is likely no one ever believed in the idols they made with their own hands. Images are, and always were, about accessing something else. Hence Latour (2002: 32) recommends a friendlier attitude to images, one that recognises the workings of the human hand as a positive asset of all images and seeks not to contain and destroy, but to provide an ever-increasing cascade of image-making.

But Latour's critique of the 'idol-haters' seems to neglect that the destruction of an image is itself also a form of mediation (Latour 2002: 17; see also Tamen 2001). Indeed, as we have seen in the previous chapter, a failed or broken image may hold a special devotional potential, residing precisely in its incapacity to represent. As Taussig (1999) points out, iconoclasm, or what he defines as 'defacement', may be a special technology for evoking and accessing the powers of the sacred. To deface an image reveals its 'sacred surplus' by showing that what was thought to be whole was only part of an excessively larger whole. As Taussig (1999: 3) writes: 'It is the cut of de/facement that releases this surplus, the cut into wholeness as holiness that, in sundering, reveals, as with film montage, not only another view via another frame, but released flows of energy.'

In the healing encounter, the nurse, psychiatrist, and shaykh listen to patients' ways of understanding and perceiving their suffering. The patient's story of the causes and manifestations of their illness is a venture into the invisible terrain of their interior. It is a visualisation of something that, as Merleau-Ponty and Levinas have taught us, in its essence cannot be made visible. Yet in these stories and images a form of self-mastering is already present. For the healers it is the task to acknowledge this, but also to produce certain fissures, so that the patients may open themselves towards the actions of the healers and the forces they represent. A form of iconoclastic overpowering is required in order to facilitate the opening or clearance through which new stories and images of the suffering within the patient can be produced. With Foucault (1982: 283; 1988: 252, 274ff) we can describe the work of the healers as the mediation of what he calls 'pastoral power' – a mode of power originating in religious institutions but which in a renewed form has also come to play a crucial role in modern psychiatry. This power does not primarily operate through repression but through pedagogical persuasion and care by making visible what is harmful to patients and where they might find healing and salvation.

Yet the healer's rendition of the suffering that occurs within the invisible terrain of patients is essentially impossible, since pain as such is always in excess. The identification of the name of the jinn or the designation of a psychiatric diagnosis is often subsequently revealed as incomplete, insufficient, or even false. For Latour such 'image-making' as an inevitable side effect of 'image-destruction' is crudely ironic. As he writes: 'Why is it that all those destroyers of images, those "theoclasts," those iconoclasts, those "ideoclasts" have also generated such a fabulous population of new images, fresh icons, rejuvenated mediators: greater flows of media, more powerful *ideas*, stronger *idols*' (2002: 17, italics in the original). Latour rightly attributes this curious phenomenon to the fact that any human being, even an iconoclast, needs mediation. Yet the iconoclasts are not necessarily unaware of the irony.

My interlocutors – if we may refer to their practices through the prism of iconoclasm – were acutely aware of what Latour describes as the danger of 'seeing oneself as a prophet'. I suggest this is why I often found both psychiatrists and Muslim healers themselves actively sowing doubt about the certainties conjured through their own imagery – acts of what, with Taussig, we could call self-defacement. As Taussig (1999: 253) states, this is a method of 'opening up', a humbling of the heart or the mind through which the images one has conjured are abolished in order to allow for the emergence of better ones. The oscillation between visibility and invisibility, certainty and doubt, image-making and image-breaking provides a destabilisation that both patients and healers must endure in order to obtain the special condition of mind that is necessary in order to let oneself be acted upon and receive this action with a stance of patience.

## The knight of faith

Feisal looks at me as I hold his knees. Erdam holds his shoulders from behind. In comes Abu Bilal carrying a glass of water. He is followed by Walid, Hassan, and Fadi – three of the young men from the mosque who have spent the night here as a religious retreat.

Abu Bilal takes my seat, puts his right hand on Feisal's chest, and starts reciting again. Instantly the body starts to shake. The spirit is back. Abu Bilal reads over the water and tries to tip it into Feisal's mouth. It looks as if most of it ends up on the floor. But sounds indicate that he is about to throw up.

Abu Bilal speaks in Arabic: 'How many are you? Get out of him.'

The guttural sounds continue. Abu Bilal threatens with more water. It works – suddenly the jinn is out. A moment of relief. Then almost immediately the jinn is replaced by another.

'How many are you?' Abu Bilal cries. He seems to be getting desperate.

At last he shifts to Danish and calls Feisal back: 'Come, Feisal, come, sit up.'

Feisal returns. He is confused and disoriented. He seems dizzy. Abu Bilal asks what he remembers. Feisal remembers that he made the sign of the cross with his hand and that he heard himself crying, but not much else.

Abu Bilal is decisive in his diagnosis: 'You have jinn, it's absolutely certain. You have many and you also have *siḥr* (magic). Two jinn came out and they became Muslims, but you need extra treatment. We need to do *ruqya* on you again.'

Feisal explains that his mother gave him protection against jinn when he was a child in Bosnia, in the form of sugar. She got it from a shaykh.

Abu Bilal says that this could have been magic: 'Many people do *siḥr* in Bosnia.'

Feisal's legs are cold and have gone to sleep, but the leg muscle is still twitching.

'Look,' says Feisal, pointing his finger at it.

Abu Bilal asks Feisal not to think too much about his lower leg. It could be the work of the jinn, but it could just as well be a nerve or a muscle. It could also be something psychological. Feisal tells Abu Bilal that his previous shaykh did not think it was jinn and told him to go to a psychologist.

'No, 100 per cent, you have jinn,' says Abu Bilal, 'but you might have a psychological problem too. Sometimes people who have jinn also get psychological problems. They think: "What's this, what's this?" But you are strong. You have many jinn, but we will get them out. You will be well again. Continue to pray.'

Abu Bilal asks if Feisal has images or music in his home. Feisal has already removed all this. Feisal says his wife has started to feel the vibrations in her leg as well.

'Don't think too much about the leg,' says Abu Bilal. 'We will get you well, you are strong, you have *īmān* [certitude or faith] … Many people work with *siḥr*, many don't have anything better to do than to harm you, they may use all their time to harm you.'

'But where's the *siḥr*, in Bosnia or here?' Feisal asks.

'It can be many places, perhaps you drank it, perhaps they have taken something from you, a hair or something and thrown a *siḥr* into the ocean, or dug it into a hole. But we'll get it. Next time we'll get it, *in shā' Allāh*.'

During the following months I learned that Feisal's jinn often attempted to drive him to suicide. According to Feisal, he still had the power to fight and control his jinn, but sometimes he could almost not continue. I was extremely uncomfortable with the situation and discussed it with Feisal, his friends, and Abu Bilal. The serious nature of the matter made me switch indecisively between Islamic, psychiatric, and anthropological modes of understanding his suffering. I tried to make Feisal see a doctor, but he refused. He had already asked a doctor about his leg. The doctor had told him to take vitamin D tablets. Of course Feisal had not told the doctor precisely what he thought was going on in his leg. It was difficult to talk to Feisal about these things. One day after another exorcism he told me that when he left the mosque to go home he often felt like a hypocrite (*munāfiq*). Sometimes he thought all these jinn were just something he made up.

Feisal's statement is serious, since hypocrisy or double-sidedness (*nifāq*) is regarded as the most dangerous illness of all. As described in Chapter 3, *nifāq* basically consists of being fully aware of the existence of the law of the divine, but secretly denying it while pretending to obey. As stated in Surat al-Baqara (Quran 2: 8–9, 14–15):

> Some people say, 'We believe in God and the Last Day,' when really they do not believe. They seek to deceive God and the believers but they only deceive themselves, though they do not realize it. [...] When they meet the believers, they say, 'We believe,' but when they are alone with their evil ones, they say, 'We're really with you; we were only mocking.' God is mocking them, and allowing them more slack to wander blindly in their insolence.

The illness of *nifāq* is infinitely more dangerous than jinn possession. While one will eventually be rewarded for the pain endured in possession if the hardship has been faced with patience, *nifāq* is never rewarded. Instead the *munāfiqūn* are severely punished: 'There is a disease in their hearts, to which God has added more: agonizing torment awaits them for their persistent lying' (Quran 2: 10).

Feisal seems desperate when he tells me of the doubts he has about his own condition. His self-perception fluctuates between a counterfeit and undisclosed experience of self-mastery, and a state of being completely in the hands of various invisible agencies; a total inability to exert self-control. His doubt, his experience of *nifāq*, and his defacement of the reality of his jinn are expressive of a deep, convoluted form of resignation that runs parallel as a contrapuntal and dissonant theme to the extreme visible outbursts of bodily dispossession that take place once he enters the altered state of *ṣarʿ*. These two poles – Feisal's claim that his lack of self-control is the will of God, and his statement that his jinn might be creations of his own – are somehow each other's conditional prerequisites.

In describing such a paradoxical oscillation between doubt and faith, Kierkegaard's De Silentio (2005: 44) distinguishes between two curious figures – the Knight of Infinite Resignation, capable only of relinquishing the visible and finite world, and the Knight of Faith, capable of grasping finitude on the strength of the absurd. In a certain way, Merleau-Ponty's phenomenology of perception can be understood in terms of these movements of resignation and faith. His whole philosophy consisted of an attempt to establish that we are indeed a part of this world. Human perception does not merely exist within us, but occurs to us through our embeddedness in the infinite web of viewpoints that surrounds us and provides the context against which objects stand out to us as visible. This is the inaccessible, yet ever-present 'view from everywhere' by which Merleau-Ponty defines the invisible (2002: 78; Kelly 2005).

Merleau-Ponty's theory of perception possibly gained its importance precisely because this co-existence and perceptual complicity between ourselves and the world seems by no means evident. Since the world – and what Merleau-Ponty refers to as the total invisible – is uncontainable, it is also inherently ambiguous. As Elisabetta Basso (2011: 249) points out in a discussion of Merleau-Ponty's inheritance from Kierkegaard, the perception of things in this world 'whose sense or meaning is neither fixed, definitive, nor guaranteed – is a form of faith'. In Kierkegaard's conception it is a faith, since it requires a paradoxical movement beyond the suggestive impression that vision can be reduced to the visible display occurring in front of our eyes (Merleau-Ponty 2002: 82; Basso 2011: 242). To perceive things as fully three-dimensional distinct objects requires faith in an invisible depth that lies beyond what we immediately see. For Merleau-Ponty, this faith operates like a natural instinct at the level of our motor-intentional actions. Yet at other levels of perception and conceptual thought, faith is, as for Kierkegaard, the site of a constant paradoxical struggle, which only a few people can overcome.[8]

In these practices of healing, are we witnessing a glimpse of the movements of faith that Kierkegaard's De Silentio was attempting to capture and describe? I believe something like this is happening when Feisal, after having gone through great measures of apparently jinn-related pain, suddenly renounces the reality of his possession as something he possibly made up. A few days later he calls me, explaining once again how the jinn are cutting in his lower legs with their knives, and asks if I can organise yet another exorcism with Abu Bilal. It also seems to occur when Abu Bilal – having just explained how psychiatric medicine is an instrument of *shayṭān* – assures me that really Aziz needs to keep taking his drugs since he is probably suffering from a multiple personality disorder. And it seems to occur just at the point when the shaykh who reportedly is the best Muslim healer in Scandinavia claims that the most important thing he does is redirect his patients to a psychiatric hospital.

Just after Jørgen has explained how the beneficial effects of psychiatric drugs are primarily derived from placebo – that is, from the faith patients and healers have in them, rather than in qualities inherent to the drugs themselves – his mobile phone rings, providing me with another example of the complexities that psychiatrists have to navigate in their work. A nurse needs Jørgen to confirm a change of medication.

'Was it Truxal she got before?' Jørgen asks. 'She needs something else to calm her thoughts. 25 milligrams of Truxal is the standard dose. You suggest she should get 1 milligram of Respidon – is that what you suggest? Try that for a month or so – see if the results are good.'

For me it is astonishing to witness how Jørgen, other psychiatrists, the nurses, shaykhs, and patients all move between denunciations and affirmations of the efficacy of biomedicine and Islamic healing practices. I see paradoxes everywhere and am brought to increasing levels of doubt, while they act as if no paradox had ever existed. Would it be these movements of faith that De Silentio describes?

This movement performed by Jørgen as he lifts the phone and prescribes Respidon – as in the perfect and impossible leap of a dancer 'straight into a definite position, so that not for a second does he have to catch at the position but stands there in it in the leap itself' (Kierkegaard 2005: 45) – is it the double movement of faith? Having first denounced the earthly causal world, having resigned from its apparent truths, the healer takes it up again as he lifts the phone, grasps this finite impossible world on the strength of the absurd.

In these communities of healers, in the psychiatric institutions, and among the shaykhs in the mosque, I feel surrounded by movements of such grace. Movements that I myself cannot make, despite how hard I try, trapped as I am by an excessive compulsive reification of doubt as the only truth. I might be capable of taking the first important step into resignation. But not that second step of the healers, having renounced their healing, they gently return to their task of healing and heal on the strength of the absurd.

As an anthropologist I have been expertly taught how impossible this world and any claim to truth about it are. Any declaration of truth sticks in the throat. As made clear by countless anthropological exercises in deconstruction, this is the world of falsity. As Kierkegaard's De Silentio (2005) points out, the very down-to-earth economic proverb 'Only one who works gets bread' is indeed odd, because it surely cannot belong to this outward world of imperfection. The psychiatrist, the nurse, and the Muslim shaykh know all too well that work in this earthly world does not by necessity result in bread.

As Jørgen points out, it is very difficult to scientifically measure a coherent, unified, positive effect for much psychiatric medicine. Critics of biomedicine point out that experiments which do seem to prove a positive effect are almost always affiliated to or sponsored by large transnational pharmaceutical companies. As Mathieu Doucet and Sergio Sismondo (2008: 627) point out, overwhelming statistical evidence shows 'a clear association between pharmaceutical industry funding of clinical trials and pro-industry results'. Also reviewing industry-sponsored psychopharmacology trials, Daniel Safer (2002: 589) comes to the same conclusion: 'those who pay the piper call the tune' (see also Healy 1997; 2001, 2006; Baker et al. 2003; Turner, Knoepflmacher, and Shapley 2012).

Nikolas Rose (2003: 46, 54) describes how in modern 'psychopharmacological' societies an additional problem is that new psychiatric illnesses (such as depression, PTSD, and anxiety or mood disorders), along with their diagnostic criteria and their biochemical treatments, are often co-produced in collaboration between psychiatric healthcare professionals, support and anti-stigma groups, and pharmaceutical companies. Often psychiatric drugs are marketed indirectly through the promotion of the illness, as with the co-funding of disease-awareness campaigns, which actively contribute to the cultivation of the kind of self that would need the drugs. Drawing on Foucault, Rose (2003: 53) identifies the particular subject taking shape in the matrix of these processes as the 'neurochemical self' – a self who attributes social and emotional dysfunctions, and the inability to satisfy the norms of autonomous self-fulfilment, to biochemical deficiencies in the brain (see also Rabinow 1996).

To my knowledge, no statistical research has been conducted on the Islamic healing practices of *ruqya shar'iyya*. Yet on the basis of the cases I have been following I suggest that such research would be extremely difficult, and might easily be subject to similar forms of bias as those applying to psychopharmacology. Even though some shaykhs demand payment for their services and many would happily accept a gift in return for their work, they are not, as the institution of modern psychiatry is, affiliated with large transnational economic interests. Yet these treatments and their advertising through sermons and lectures, book publications, webpages, and YouTube videos are also aimed at cultivating a particular kind of self that could hardly be conceived of without such illnesses constantly threatening its moral integrity. The threats represented by *shayṭān*, magic, and the world of the jinn call for further measures of Quranic healing, purification, and prayer, hence cultivating increasingly more advanced ways of disciplining and fortifying the pious Muslim self.

However, regardless of these seemingly self-fulfilling mechanisms, shaykhs often experience that their Quranic readings do not work as powerfully as they should. Furthermore, critics abound within Muslim communities arguing for or against the possibility of jinn interfering in the world of humankind. Stories and accusations of fraudsters masquerading as shaykhs are also frequent. One day after Friday prayers Abu Bilal addressed his community and issued a warning against a Sufi shaykh from one of the other mosques who, apparently under the pretext of healing, had begun to insert jinn into the breasts of his female patients. Abu Bilal had received several cases of such miserable women who had become severely ill after attending a healing session with this shaykh. I did not do fieldwork in this mosque and so I have no way of verifying these accusations, but I could imagine that very similar claims addressed in the opposite direction could well be made with regard to the activities of the neo-orthodox Muslims with whom I worked.

All of this goes to say that healing in the Muslim communities, as in psychiatric healthcare, is a highly disputed and contested endeavour. The field and its practitioners are subject to intense scrutiny, scepticism, slander, and valuation. Regardless of how doctrinal both psychiatric healthcare and Islamic healing might appear on the surface, there simply is no consensus. Despite claims to objective knowledge, the truth is always deferred into the realm of the invisible. In this way the truth acts like the inaccessible norm described by Merleau-Ponty, from which all partial claims and perspectives are derived and evaluated.

Shaykhs, as well as nurses and psychiatrists, frequently express doubts arising from the brute indifference that characterises the tangible effects of their healing methods. These doubts that healers in both systems have about their healing are, however, not merely 'matter out of place' (Douglas 2002). As also demonstrated in Lévi-Strauss's (1993[1963]) classic study of the 'Sorcerer and his Magic', doubt appears to be a recurrent issue for healers and patients in many different cultural traditions (see also Severi 2002; Pelkmans 2013). I therefore propose, following Kierkegaard, that doubt is integral to the act of faith required by healing. Indeed doubt is its facilitating obstacle, a kind of fuel that makes the leap into faith more difficult and threatening, yet infinitely more rewarding. If it is not there, it must be produced through acts of defacement and iconoclastic destruction.

In psychiatry, the industry appears to take an active part in the production of doubt and the defacement of its products, as seen for example in the extensive lists of side effects that expose, among other curious malaises, how antipsychotic medication and antidepressants may at times produce even greater degrees of psychosis and depression (Rose 2003: 55). Somehow the scarring and calling into question of the individual case allows for an even greater, more powerful truth to be evoked, the truth as deferred into the realm of the invisible. As Taussig (1999: 12–13, 249) makes clear, this 'labour of the negative' is a decidedly mystical process, through which defacement and resignation somehow lead to faithful 'refacement' and thereby the release of even further degrees of sacred potential.

The healing movements of these practitioners by no means lie in a simple, mechanical passing on of external agents, psychotropics, or Quranic words. Rather, their function is to provide a specific mediation between the invisible and the visible, so that these external agents are inserted into the patient through procedures invested with full conviction and pure intention – *ikhlāṣ*, as it would be termed in the Islamic context – that they will heal. It does not seem enough for the psychiatrist, nurse, or shaykh to simply carry out the procedures. In the act of doing them, they must do them in full faith of their efficacy. Faith and certitude, as De Silentio points out, imply a double, paradoxical movement – namely resignation from the finite world and grasping it again on the strength of the absurd.

With Kierkegaard's De Silentio, I suggest that what these healers do is to invite their patients along with them on the path towards the acceptance and therefore the overcoming of this paradox – recognising the absurd, opaque, and contingent character of the world, yet perceiving it and acting in it as if it was in fact capable of being correctly perceived. A paradox of this sort is not resolved through logical reasoning (see also Merleau-Ponty 1976). Rather, it is resolved by embracing and submitting to it as such. By embracing the paradox, an opening is facilitated through which the submission of the patient to the external agencies of psychotropics, placebo, or God is made possible.

It may appear as if what the shaykhs, psychiatrists, and nurses do in the instance of healing is a form of dissimulation, an active, consciously deployed form of 'false consciousness' – a forgetting of certain things in order to attend fully to their practice (Taussig 1993).[9] Yet with the aid of Merleau-Ponty, De Silentio, and Kierkegaard we can take a different view. Namely that the remarkable manoeuvre of the healers is not so much to forget the impossibility of finitude, full visibility, or the lack of evidential proof for healing. Rather, I suggest what they do is simply not to demand that their healing efforts need to be rewarded in the realm of finitude. These healers have already 'drained in infinite resignation', as Kierkegaard would phrase it, and thereby learned the virtues of patience. Only in this way, by actively facing and recognising the impossibility of the visible, finite world, are they able to embrace it by taking a leap of faith. In other words, it is not by forgetting the paradox that these forms of healing become possible; if the healer and the patient had simply forgotten the paradox, we could not speak of submission or what in psychiatric language is sometimes called 'compliance'. Their acting in the world as if it was not impossible would not have been absurd, only naive. Compliance and submission are facilitated precisely because of the existence of a paradox and its overcoming by faith. Within both psychiatric and neo-orthodox Islamic practices, healing begins once this opening towards the realm of the invisible – *al-ghayb*, God, psychotropics, and placebo – is established.

The concept 'patient' is related to patience, the ability to inhabit the space of pain, the capacity of letting oneself be moved by something beyond one's own control. Agency as used in much current anthropological writing is related to certainty, knowledge, and vision, as without a path for action, agency is blind and powerless. The form of healing pursued in both the religious and psychiatric treatments I studied seems to involve a dismantling of certainties, common-sense perceptions, and ideas for agentive action. To become a patient one needs uncertainty, in order to then overcome uncertainty through faith. In this healers invite their patients to join a set of movements they themselves are also oscillating between. These movements involve disbelieving one's own taken-for-granted perceptions so as to move beyond the limits of resignation, thereby allowing the external healing agents to do their work.

## Notes

1 Ibn Qayyim al-Jawziyah (2003: 69) describes the state of *ṣarʿ* in his book on prophetic medicine (see also Badeen and Krawietz 2003: 103). While the word *ruqya* is customarily used to denote lawful Quranic incantations, Pandolfo (2011: 32; 2018: 265) describes how the word literally refers to 'spiritual elevation'.

2 Pierre Bourdieu's (1977) theory of practice can be understood as an attempt at bridging these two notions of agency. However, while Bourdieu with his concept of 'habitus' mainly emphasises how social structures and class positions are reproduced through the embodiment of largely unconcious dispositions for action, Mahmood and Asad focus on highly conscious attempts to cultivate the self through virtuous conduct (for a discussion see Mahmood 2005: 136).

3 In Danish the word 'imam' is often used instead of 'shaykh' to designate a Muslim of religious authority.

4 In a discussion of aniconic, Islamic art, Marks (2010: 49–53) argues against the commonly held idea 'that Islam is categorically opposed to images' by showing how images of all kinds have populated the history of art in the Muslim world. Yet, in accordance to what Abu Bilal claims here, Marks points out how aniconism is part of a critique of 'spiritual mediation … that asserts the abstraction, ineffability, and unknowability – but also the beauty and goodness – of God'.

5 These developments are in opposition to the early psychiatric interventions described by Foucault (1988: 264) aiming to make the 'madman' recognise 'himself as objectively mad'. They also appear to contradict Merleau-Ponty's (2002: 107) understanding of pain and suffering as always occuring on the side of 'me'. Many interventions in contemporary Danish psychiatry, such as cognitive behavioral therapy, work to relieve patients from pain by helping them to identify the patterns of thinking and behaving that reinforce their distress so that these patterns may be replaced by alternative ways of thinking and behaving.

6 James C. Scott's (1990) notions of 'hidden' and 'public transcripts' are useful for understanding the complex interaction between Aziz and Esther. Sometimes what is 'hidden' and what is 'public' shifts in unexpected and contradictory ways.

7 Such an opinion was also expressed by the influential Egyptian shaykh Yusuf al-Qaradawi. See e.g. https://archive.islamonline.net/?p=1408 (retrieved 27 September 2017).

8 In this lies both Kierkegaard and Merleau-Ponty's criticism of the late G.W. F. Hegel. Against Hegel's claim that eventually comprehending the absolute through dialectical reasoning is a human possibility, Merleau-Ponty (1976; Basso 2011: 250) posits what we with Taussig could call a defaced philosophical attitude of 'non-philosophy'. The absolute, or what Merleau-Ponty defines as the infinite 'view from everywhere', is invisible, and indeed it must remain invisible in order for any of our partial viewpoints to be possible. According to Merleau-Ponty (1988: 5), what we should seek to acquire is not absolute knowledge, 'but its becoming in us … our absolute relation to it, as Kierkegaard said'.

9 Taussig's concepts of 'defacement' and 'refacement' lies in continuation of his work on the mimetic faculty, in which he describes how the capacity for dissimulation involves an active forgetting of what was dissimulated in the first place (see Taussig 1993). By this mysterious process the deceiver slips into her or his own fiction, which then becomes believed in as fact. Taussig points out that such active forgetting of the fundamentally constructed character of the social fact is indeed what makes social life possible (Taussig 1993: xvii; 1999). The concept of dissimulation offers the possibility that what was originally fantasy and fiction might, if it proves useful and desirable, take on a reality of its own and through reification become felt as really real. Even though Taussig shows the enormous potential inherent in the act of defacement, we should keep in mind that for Taussig the power of this always and necessarily deferred truth rests purely in its falsity. For Taussig (1999: 7), the great

'public secret' is that 'there is no such thing as a secret'. Hence Taussig operates within what we could call a flat ontology. This is not so for my interlocutors in the mosques and in the psychiatric institutions. Regardless of their repeated acts of defacement, they live their lives in a decidedly deep ontology in which truth can by no means be disregarded. It is certainly there, yet always deferred and inaccessible to our view.

5

# Healing through sacrifice

*He said: 'O my son! I have seen in a dream that I am slaughtering you, so look what you think!'*

*He said: 'O my father! Do that which you are commanded, God willing, you shall find me of the patient and persevering ones.' Then, when they had both submitted themselves (to the Will of God), and he had laid him prostrate on his forehead; And We called out to him: 'O Abraham! You have fulfilled the dream!' Verily! Thus do We reward the good-doers. Verily, that indeed was a manifest trial. And We ransomed him with a great sacrifice; And We left for him (a goodly remembrance) among generations in later times. 'Peace be upon Abraham!' Thus indeed do We reward the good-doers. Verily, he was one of Our believing slaves.*

Quran, Surat al-Saffat (102–11)

## Making sacred

In a seminal article from 1987, Thomas Csordas takes issue with the ways in which medical anthropologists have often analysed religious or spiritual practices as indigenous forms of psychotherapy (see e.g. Kiev 1962; Edgerton 1971; Crapanzano 1973; Pattison 1977; Kleinman 1980). Csordas calls for a greater focus on the commonalities between 'medical' and 'religious' approaches to healing, but it is not just that religious aspects of healing should be understood 'emically' as opposed to an 'etic' understanding of the medical aspects. Rather, Csordas (1987: 1) argues that: 'scientific accounts can be formulated of religious phenomena qua religious, as well as in clinical terms'. Indeed in cross-cultural studies of healing, the 'sacred' might be of equal importance to such medical categories as 'disease' and 'illness'. Discussing a variety of African and Afro-American cases of spirit possession, Csordas argues that to the extent we may be inclined to see spirit possession as an idiom for understanding certain exotic ways of dealing with illness, we should to the same extent be ready to see illness as an idiom for encounters with the sacred. Hence Csordas (*ibid.*) concludes that a complete account of healing 'must not only examine the construction of clinical reality with respect to medical motives, but also the construction of sacred reality with respect to religious motives'.

This book and film examine the similarities and differences between how healing is pursued and understood in psychiatric healthcare and by

Muslim shaykhs in Denmark. A key insight of my research has been to discover the ways in which the 'sacred' and what, with Merleau-Ponty, Levinas, and Kierkegaard, I have referred to as the 'invisible' play a role in both Islamic exorcisms as well as in psychiatric healthcare.

In a similar way, the anthropologist Sjaak van der Geest (2005) has called for an anthropology of the spiritual and ritual dimensions of modern medicine. Hospitals can easily be taken as places of secularisation on the fringes of life. Despite the fact that religion often becomes important during illness, religious agents have almost become matter out of place in modern hospitals. As van der Geest (2005: 135) observes, it may appear as if '[m]edical scientists and technicians have taken over the role of priests and other religious specialists in times of crisis and in the face of death'. Yet he notices how medical words and interventions work in strikingly 'religious' ways to express and recreate people's belief in science and biomedicine as an 'ultimate truth'. However, van der Geest's study is by no means an attempt to belittle the therapeutic efficacy of biomedicine. Rather, he aims to show how the work of magic and religious sacraments need to be considered in order for the proper mechanics of biomedical recovery to be understood (see also Nathan and Stengers 2018).

My analysis here takes its cue from Csordas and van der Geest's invitation to upturn the distinctions between what is often regarded as belonging to the sacred and to the medical. Not only is the 'medical' a problematic concept, indeed the 'sacred' is equally problematic. As pointed out by Asad (2003: 29), the history of the 'sacred' as the antonym of the 'profane' is closely associated with the rise of the modern secular. Therefore we need to ask which ways of being human are enabled or disabled within a social formation that has been built around such terms.

The 'sacred', in its classical sense as derived from Latin, simply refers to anything owned by a deity, including the area surrounding a temple (Fowler 1920: 15; Asad 2003: 30). If with Csordas and van der Geest we accept the idea that both modern medical healthcare and neo-orthodox Islamic practices of exorcism facilitate encounters with the sacred, then we need to ask what the sacred is constituted by; who are the divinities worshipped by these forms of practice? In the Islamic case it is quite clearly Allah, the almighty God who in numerous supplications is referenced as the only deity worthy of worship, a continuously deferred divinity, always greater than any human utterance could contain.

In the psychiatric case it is more complicated, but the primary reference is science and more particularly biomedicine (van der Geest 2005; Petryna and Kleinman 2006; Rose 2018). As already indicated in previous chapters, psychiatrists, and especially psychiatric nurses, do not always appear consistent in their devotional practices, and it is not clear whether their frequent acts of criticism and defacement really do lead to a deferred 'refacement' of the truth of science and biomedicine – a problem I address in the last chapter of this book. But let us, at least for now and for the sake of this analysis, stick to the idea that biomedicine as manifested in the tangible form of psychotropic drugs is the primary deity worshipped in Danish psychiatric healthcare. This is precisely the conclusion reached by many of my Muslim interlocutors. As pointed out by Aziz in Scene 3: 'The doctors don't believe in jinn, the Quran, or the imam, they don't believe in anything, only medicine.'

How are encounters with the sacred facilitated? How is something evoked as sacred in the therapeutics of Danish psychiatry and in Islamic exorcisms? In the following paragraphs I will consider practices of 'making sacred' through the idiom of sacrifice (Carter 2003: 2). Keeping to the original sense of the sacred, we can understand 'making sacred' simply as the moving of something into the domain of the gods. Sacrifice then is the giving or returning of something to the gods (Hubert and Mauss 1964). This minimal definition makes good sense considering the Islamic concept *qurbān*, used to describe Abraham's sacrifice of the ram at the mountain of Moriah – the offer that later came to serve as the model for the animal sacrifices performed each year at the Islamic feast of *'Īd al-aḍḥā*.

Yet sacrifice as an active gesture is difficult to imagine when dealing with an almighty divinity who is at once the creator, controller, and destroyer of everything. In this context sacrifice is not so much a matter of giving an amount of meat or blood to a divinity, but rather of acknowledging and making visible that whatever is sacrificed is in fact already in the possession of the divinity. As stated in Surat al-Hajj (Quran 22: 37): 'It is not their meat nor their blood that reaches God: it is your piety that reaches Him.' If the 'sacred' cannot be distinguished as a realm beyond this world but is at once the origin, cause, and endpoint of everything, then piety becomes a matter of recognising and acknowledging one's inevitable state of dependency, that one is already in the hands of the 'sacred'; that there is no outside, no escape from the space and rulings of divine law. What is sacrificed then is the illusion of one's personal autonomy, entitlement, and perceptual mastery.

Sacrifice has long divided debates in social theory. Theologians and philosophers such as Edward Kessler (2004) and Sidney Axinn (2010) have emphasised the intrinsic value of sacrifice as an act of faith and gesture of unconditional commitment to the divine. This was also the view of George Bataille (1991[1967]), who described sacrifice as the absolute profitless destruction of surplus value with no expectation of material gain. According to Bataille, both the sacrificial victim and the sacrificer 'withdraw from the real order' and find a momentary escape from the 'cold calculation' of the general economy by negating any utilitarian relationship (Bataille 1991: 60; see also Carter 2003). In contrast to this, anthropologists such as Henri Hubert and Marcel Mauss (1964), Evans-Pritchard (1956), and Maurice Bloch (1992) have provided different perspectives by emphasising the utility and instrumental value of sacrifice as the act of giving something in exchange for something of greater value.

Willerslev (2013b) summarises this long-standing debate and argues that the co-presence of seemingly contradictory 'instrumental' and 'intrinsic' values is, in fact, crucial for the workings of sacrifice. In this he points to the necessity of a paradoxical tension, paralleling the enigmatic absurdity of faith as described by Kierkegaard. However, in the presence of an almighty divinity, such as those evoked by the laws of biomedical science or the Islamic God, there is no escape from the sacred, and thus there can be no contradiction between the intrinsic and instrumental values of sacrifice. Rather, sacrifice becomes generalised as a constant struggle of the self (*jihād al-nafs*) to acknowledge the absolute ruling of divine law, letting oneself submit to it as the only agent that could ever provide shelter from the misfortunes of life (see also Foucault 1988: 262, 275). This is not the escape from the general economy of which Bataille writes. Rather, as Pandolfo (2007: 344–6) describes with reference to the Iranian philosopher Ali Shariati's (1979) understanding of martyrdom, sacrifice is a witnessing (*shahāda*) and expression of trust (*tawakkul*) in the fact that the economy, like everything else, is also taking place within the jurisdiction of the divine. It is an act of faith, but not in contradiction to any form of instrumental act, since faith in the divine doctrine is acknowledged through sacrifice as the principal instrument for addressing the powers that may relieve one's suffering. Sacrifice, in other words, is an instrumental attempt to escape the rule of jinn, psychotic delusions, or other false sovereignties of an earthly origin – thereby aligning oneself with the divine by expressing one's faith in its ultimate and universal application.

It may seem odd to suggest that sacrifice should have anything to do with healing, as sacrifice seems to imply some form of violence or transgression. How precisely is this related to the Islamic and psychiatric treatments I studied in Denmark?

## Trance is a violation of the ego

Abu Bilal is sitting on the chair behind Nadia, the Bosnian woman in Scene 5. On her own initiative, she has put on an improvised veil for the occasion. During her previous conversation with the shaykh she preferred not to wear the veil, but now it is time to attend to the healing words of the Quran. The Arabic word for veil is *ḥijāb* – commonly identified as a piece of cloth used to cover the head. Yet in the Quran, the *ḥijāb* also has the more general connotation of a barrier or screen between the visible world and those parts of reality that are not supposed to be visible (Quran 42: 51; see also Pandolfo 1997: 240 and Chapter 1). As the full display of a woman is not supposed to be revealed to a man before marriage, so the future and the unseen are not to be shown before it is exposed by God. This insistency on invisibility is also why fortune telling and other forms of visionary practice are strictly condemned within neo-orthodox Islam. Indeed some of my interlocutors reported that a single glance into the future by way of newspaper horoscopes may render a full month of prayer invalid.

When Nadia puts on the veil in this context of Islamic healing we may understand it either in positive terms, as a gesture of modesty, or more negatively, as a giving in to the pressure of the religious norms embodied by the shaykh.[1] It is also, however, a physical expression of the fact that whatever goes on within her cannot be fully understood or grasped from a human perspective. It lies beyond our gaze within the realm of the invisible. The figure of the healer is ambiguous in this context, as he claims to be able to know and see into the suffering reported by the patient, while at the same time he is obviously and literally unable to see. The 'image-breaker' who just a few minutes ago took down the photographs and drawing in his patient's bedroom, is now on the verge of becoming an 'image-maker' (Latour 2002: 16).

Abu Bilal starts to recite the Quran. For several minutes nothing seems to happen, but then small movements begin to appear. Just a faint shaking. I move my camera to get a better perspective. The movements stop. Was it me who interrupted? I feel distracted by my own movement. I am unsure if it has also interrupted the interaction between Nadia and the shaykh. Abu Bilal continues to recite. His voice gets louder and the speed of the recitation intensifies. The whole room appears to vibrate. Nadia starts to shiver again. When Abu Bilal reads Surat al-Baqara, she joins in with the recitation and begins to cry. After approximately twenty minutes the reading ends. Abu Bilal gives his diagnosis: Nadia is definitely not possessed by a jinn, but she might have been stroked by one.

Jørgen asks me to pause the video of Abu Bilal and Nadia (Scene 6). He has a question: 'I would like to ask, is this a regular liturgy [*fast messetekst*]?'

I reply that they are verses from the Quran.

'Who understands this, it's nicely translated,' Jørgen asks.

'By now, I know most of these verses,' I reply, 'it's specific verses from the Quran they use.'

'And does the girl understand it?' Jørgen asks.

'I don't think she understands everything, she doesn't speak Arabic, but she probably understands half of it. And then she would know the larger part of it, but not necessarily so that she would understand each word.'

Esther enters the discussion: 'But she knows the content?'

I confirm: 'Yes, at least the key pieces – but perhaps not 100 per cent because she doesn't speak Arabic.'

Jørgen: 'But it is a liturgy, a canonised text?'

'Yes, it is recognised as some of the most forceful texts for exorcisms.'

Then Jørgen presents his analysis:

'What I notice is that he speaks with his own mouth, he doesn't speak with the mouth of God. This is a very important detail, in my opinion, because in many other religions you have your eyes in the text.'

Jørgen picks up his block of paper and looks at it.

'You speak with the mouth of God because it is God … who has written the text, so to speak. Therefore you are not a subject – well, you are – but you are a transmission of it – therefore you have your eyes in the text. This is very important in many religions. But I noticed that he didn't. The other thing which is very characteristic in many religions is that one doesn't understand what is being said. In the Christian Church it was Latin, right, until I don't know when. One didn't understand the mass, nobody understands the mass. So then they understand the sound of the mass.

'They don't understand every word,' I add.

'No, far from it.' Jørgen continues: 'They can read the text in [Latin] or their own language. This I also think is interesting, because is the Quran translated into the languages of the world?'

'Yes, it is,' I reply.

Jørgen: 'Well, okay. But the mass in the Church, everywhere in the Catholic Church the mass is in Latin, and no one understands it, but they understand the melody.'

At this point in the discussion I start to sense where Jørgen is going. I decide to emphasise that Nadia has a good understanding of most of what goes on: 'She has most probably read the Quran in translation, and she's also able to recite some of the verses on her own – you can see it on her lips. But she probably doesn't understand that it is this exact word which has that meaning. But is there a particular function in this?'

Jørgen explains: 'You get the other human being into a trance – partly through the melody, partly through the repetition, one doesn't need to understand it, it's the very tone, because by constantly maintaining the tone, something else is kept out – that is, in the head of the patient, the human being. When something else is kept out of the human being then you can induce trance through this path.'

'It's like a mantra,' Esther adds.

Jørgen continues: 'This is why I am very concerned about whether she understands it or not because the power is much greater in just repeating the same, using the same melody, you know what I mean, because it's the setting that conjures the trance. In the trance you get hold of different things, you can get in contact with everything, but you get in contact with something. Then there are differences between how fragile [*sprøde*] people are, how easily they get hypnotised. But what is characteristic is that it provides clearing [*klaring*] for the one who is in it: a catharsis, a relief. Why? Perhaps it gives a relief, but this is because the mind in fact gets purified by it, this is why it's called catharsis, the mind is purified by being under such influence [*påvirkning*]. What is important is the very setting which conjures it [*fremmer det*], you don't need to understand what is being said.'

I ask: 'So it's the very tone and the atmosphere which work as a sort of forced meditation.'

Jørgen: 'Yes, this is correct. Meditation is different because there you need yourself actively to think of something. Here it's the power from outside – that is, the priest – who puts you into a condition of exaltation. In psychiatry some people can't stand this. But some think it's enjoyable – that it produces peace of mind. And it does give peace of mind … This is the summoning [*fremkaldelse*] of a trance – it corresponds to the concept of hypnosis. A trance is summoned. And if you are a little psychologically vulnerable, you can get ill through a trance.'

Ester: 'This is what we see.'

Jørgen: 'This is what we say.'

Jørgen repeats Esther's sentence, thinking she is disagreeing with his statement. He adds: 'But we are not fully certain, right?'

'Yes, this is what we see,' Esther repeats her first sentence.

Jørgen laughs: 'Yes, this is what we see. One can become ill through trance. It's a violation [*overgreb*].'

Ester: 'I've often experienced patients who have been seeking this. In our culture they would turn to the Pentecostal Church for example.'

Jørgen: 'It gives peace [*det giver ro*]. So in psychiatry, meditation is distinguished from trance. And this is not only us, who do so. And we find that it's a little problematic with the other thing when it becomes transgressive [*grænseoverskridende*]. The reason that this has something to do with psychiatry, is that most psychiatric patients are what is called weak egos [*jeg-svage*]. Their defence is weak. For this reason they are more vulnerable when they are exposed to something which for them is experienced as transgressive … A psychiatric patient is more vulnerable to a condition where hypnosis is promoted [*fremmet*], a condition of exaltation through such a mass.'

Esther asks Jørgen: 'Could we, speaking in popular terms, say that they also have problems finding themselves again afterwards?'

'Yes, they do,' Jørgen replies, 'and this is because the ego boundaries of the psychiatric patient are weaker than others. Much weaker … People with psychological illnesses have weaker boundaries, a weaker structure of the self, they get more easily affected by such an ecstasy and trance, and as Esther says they may have difficulties finding their own selves again.'

Jørgen and Esther launch a critique of Islamic practices of exorcism, pointing to the fact that they may be harmful to patients with a weak sense of self. Key to their critique is their conception of how the ego may be transgressed by the external manipulation of Quranic recitation. On the contrary, Jørgen and Esther understand the essence of their own work as consisting in a fortification and strengthening of the boundaries of the patient's ego.

Jørgen and Esther's critique is well grounded. Several examples were related to me by nurses of Muslim patients whose families or who themselves had refused psychiatric medication and instead sought healing through exorcisms in various parts of the Middle East. After a while they would return to the psychiatric institutions, but with even greater trauma from violent – sometimes physically violent – encounters with Muslim shaykhs. Jørgen and Esther's worries about exorcisms getting out of hand are further supported by several incidents in France, Belgium, England, and throughout the Middle East, where patients have been allegedly killed by shaykhs trying to physically beat the jinn out of their bodies (see e.g. Philips 2007: 200; Drieskens 2008: 195ff; Daily Mail 2011, 2012; BBC News 2012; Huffington Post 2012). In these instances, the egos of patients are not only violated, but entirely eradicated.

However, it is clearly not only Muslim shaykhs who risk the health of their patients during acts of healing. Nurses related how it was not always straightforward to determine whether a patient was being remedied or harmed by psychotropic medication, since the side effects – such as the risk of developing diabetes, dementia, chronic headaches, 'neuroleptic induced anguish', or 'unknown sudden death' – are sometimes more dangerous than the illness itself.

Much research and literature supports the ambiguity expressed by the healthcare professionals I worked with. As Marc De Hert et al. (2010: 73) assert, most evidence from randomised clinical trials supports a beneficial effect of antipsychotics on risk of suicide, but the data also shows that many antipsychotics result in a marked increase of cardiovascular morbidity and mortality (see also Ray et al. 2009). In a study of treatment with antidepressants and the risk of suicide, Jari Tiihonen et al. (2006: 1358) came to an equally ambiguous conclusion: 'the current use of any antidepressant was associated with a markedly increased risk of attempted suicide and, at the same time, with a markedly decreased risk of completed suicide and death.' In a comparison of a large number of FDA trials, the highly industry-critical physician David Healy (2006: 70, 77; see also 1997, 2002) argues more pessimistically that in fact all available antidepressants and antipsychotics result in a marked increase in suicide. Yet this stands in contrast to much of the published literature in which, according to Healy, the risk of suicide is significantly downplayed. Healy (2006: 68) attributes the difference between clinical trials and the conclusions reached in published articles to the effect of industry-sponsored ghost writing and a general silencing of criticism in the biomedical field.

Nevertheless, criticisms such as those raised in Healy's study quickly feed into public media, newspapers, and television, fuelling the age-old anxiety about being exploited by charlatans and quacks impersonating healers for the sake of economic benefit. When I began my fieldwork for this project, the Danish newspaper *Politiken* launched a series of articles criticising the massive use of psychotropic medication both within and outside the psychiatric system (see e.g. Drachman and Goos 2012; Simonsen 2012; Schmidt 2013).

The criticisms were challenged in 2018 when *The Lancet* published the results of a large meta-analysis of the efficacy of twenty-one antidepressant drugs that aimed to put the doubts about the medicine to rest (Cipriani et al. 2018). The study generated headlines in public media such as 'The drugs do work' and 'It's official: antidepressants are not snake oil or a conspiracy' (*The Guardian*, Boseley 2018; Rice-Oxley 2018; *Politiken*, Rasmussen 2018). Immediately critics disputed these conclusions as being based on a limited evaluation of efficacy measured over eight weeks, for ignoring long-term 'real world' studies that do not confirm the reported efficacy, and for minimising the implications of the fact that the drugs are not effective in children. Critics also pointed out that these findings have no relevance to the vast majority who are receiving the drugs for the treatment of mild to moderate depression (see Rose 2018: 213 for these and additional criticisms).

For health professionals working in the psychiatric field, these criticisms and anxieties form part of their daily work. In a moment of disillusion, a nurse told me that in fact she believed her patients' lifespan was reduced by as much as twenty years on average due to the various side effects of drugs she administered. While both Quranic exorcisms and psychiatric medication are intended to heal, it is clear that there are real, tangible risks involved in both forms of healing.

This was expressed to me most directly by Abu Samir, who voiced the opinion that it is the Danish system that 'drags people down'. After he himself was subjected to treatment for depression and stress, he came to the conclusion that the treatment was inflicting a new illness upon him. What he realised was that the biomedical treatment was targeted at dampening his emotional faculties. He saw this as being part of the overall effort of the psychiatric system and the state to transform his Arab identity into being more Danish. For Abu Samir this is an impossible operation that will inevitably result in trauma. As a former psychiatric patient himself, he expresses how what he regards as the kernel of his being – his 'ego' if you like – had been under siege and was violated through psychiatric treatment.

Aziz's wife Liliane also expresses this view. After we watched a rough cut of the film together she explained how she often found her husband dimmed by psychiatric medication, which made proper Quranic treatment difficult: 'The medicine reacts against the *ruqya* … If someone who has jinn gets this medicine, he becomes apathetic. His brain stops functioning and the jinn doesn't come out when the shaykh reads the Quran. A shaykh from Lebanon told us that Aziz needed to stop his medication before he could do the *ruqya*.'

In this, Liliane counters the view of Aziz's psychiatrist Jørgen when he claims that the recitation of *ruqya* provokes a state of trance that is potentially dangerous to the patient. Liliane makes clear that *ruqya* is used not only in the treatment of jinn possession, but on an everyday basis for a variety of purposes, including small fevers, headaches, and wounds: 'If you read the Quran for someone who hasn't got a jinn then nothing happens, no trance occurs.' Furthermore she states that it is not the patient who is hurt by the Quranic reading, but the jinn. Usually the patient will not even remember the treatment. If the *ruqya* is addressed to the jinn, then it is the jinn who suffers. For this reason Liliane also objected when, in Scene 6, Jørgen argues that it is the tone and setting which provokes the trance, and that it is easier for the healer to induce trance if the patient does not understand the words of the incantation. According to Liliane the patient does not need to understand Arabic because it is the jinn and not the patient who is being addressed by the healer.

Abu Bilal made the same point when we watched a preliminary version of the film. However, as both Liliane and Abu Bilal emphasise, it is better if the patient understands and believes in the divine words. In his weekly lessons in the mosque, Abu Bilal constantly urges the mosque participants to spend more of their time practising their reading skills and understanding of the Quran. He stresses how in fact the Quran is a remedy for everything, but if people doubt its truth-value, then nothing good will be obtained from the reading: 'God's words are a healing for the illnesses of the heart, the devils' whispering, the catastrophes, the jinn, the magic, and the evil eye, the anxiety, the irritation, the illusions – it's a healing for all things. For depression it's also a healing. God confirms that the Quran is a healing. But if you don't accept this, it doesn't heal you' (see Scene 10).

In this, Abu Bilal comes close to Jørgen and Esther's explanation of placebo as a kind of 'self-healing' operating through the hope of the patient that the medication will heal them (see also Harrington 2000b: 222ff). Yet for Abu Bilal it is not faith as such that heals. Rather it is the lack of faith that prevents the patient's access to healing.

Like nurses and psychiatrists, Muslim shaykhs also discuss the possible risks inherent in various forms of healing. If a shaykh is not strong and consistent in his faith, the chances increase that the jinn will fool the shaykh, which may have fatal consequences for both patient and healer. Before undertaking any form of exorcism, a shaykh needs to be well trained in Quranic recitation and highly skilled in various other religious disciplines.

But even though the shaykhs are aware of the risks involved in exorcisms, they do not at all agree that Quranic recitation constitutes a transgressive attack on the self. Like Jørgen and Esther, they see their practices as essentially targeted at the fortification of a part of the self. But their understanding of what constitutes a healthy self is, as we shall see, somewhat different.

For now it is sufficient to say that healing in psychiatric healthcare, as well as in the mosques, seems to operate through diverse practices ultimately aimed at the fortification and strengthening of a part of the self, yet also including highly transgressive actions that verge on the destruction of other parts of the self. Common to both practices of healing is that something within the patient needs to be overpowered, removed, or surrendered in order for what is recognised as the kernel of the self to thrive again. Healers regard this violence as a fortification of the self, but for the patients it is often experienced as highly transgressive, since they are being asked to surrender something they see as essential to their way of being in the world. It is from this point of view that we can speak of healing as involving a sacrifice – the surrender of consciousness to the governing of the divine. To the extent that healers succeed in convincing the patient to surrender, we can speak of a kind of self-sacrifice. The importance of transgressive or sacrificial violence in these acts of healing leads us back to Kierkegaard's De Silentio and his concern with the near-sacrifice of Abraham's son on the mountain of Moriah.

## Sacrificing agency

What thoughts went through Abraham's mind when he stood on the mountain with his knife ready to offer up his son? Kierkegaard's De Silentio struggles throughout his book to grasp the emotional state of Abraham and his son at this moment at the summit and during the three and a half days they spent together climbing uphill to the summit. Did Isaac know of his father's project during the ascent? Did he see the blade? Could the father hide his thoughts from him? What words would have been uttered between them on this journey to Moriah?

Preparing to kill one's own son must, as Kierkegaard's De Silentio (2005: 21–3) argues, be equally terrifying or perhaps even worse than killing oneself. It is the killing of one's earthly continuation after death, the killing of compassion, and of that which constituted one's human identity as a parent. What Abraham did, De Silentio concludes, was to set aside all of what he held dearest in this world in order to carry out the divine command – to submit to it unconditionally while being fully conscious of how counterintuitive, absurd, and essentially unethical it was. De Silentio argues that Abraham did not for a split second doubt the divine command, because had he done so, his task would have become impossible. Hence he held within himself the full knowledge of the terrible act he was about to commit, but he continued, since he knew beyond all doubt that this was what he had been demanded to do. As we know, just before the sacrifice was made, God intervened. Having first given up his son, Abraham now receives him again by being allowed to substitute the ultimate sacrifice with the sacrifice of a ram. For Kierkegaard's De Silentio (2005: 55), receiving his son again was the result of that impossible move called faith – a form of certitude or obedience to God's claim on the finite and visible world, which does not appear to comply with any earthly reality, but which still persists and grasps this world as if nothing could be easier.

What is powerfully expressed by the story of Abraham is the idea that sometimes the renewal of life necessitates a sacrifice – sometimes the highest sacrifice – of that which one holds most dear (see also Willerslev 2009b). In the Islamic version this is also emphasised. Here some of De Silentio's questions regarding the actual occurrence of the event are explicated. First of all, it is clear in the Islamic version that Abraham's son was in fact well aware of his father's project.[2] Abraham received the message from God in a dream and then told this dream to his son. Thereupon the son asked his father to take him to Moriah as a sacrifice: 'God willing, you shall find me of the patient and persevering ones' (Quran 37: 102). In the Islamic version both the son and the father are complicit in the violent act that seems to entirely transgress ethical law – suicide, manslaughter, killing of one's son etc. But through this, by submitting to the divine command, life is made possible again. Earthly existence is suspended, so to speak, as a condition of its return.

It may seem far-fetched to apply this age-old model of sacrifice to the healing practices of psychiatrists, nurses, and shaykhs, but I believe it highlights key aspects of their interactions. First and foremost there is the emphasis on violence: a certain violent, transgressive, and sacrificial act is necessary for patients to be healed. Something is causing the suffering, and for the suffering to cease and the life of the patient to be resumed, this something needs to be done away with. Yet much common-sense wisdom and immediate intuition would suggest that violence cannot be healing. Indeed on the surface of things it seems to be a hurting rather than a caring that the patient undergoes when the Quran is read loudly into their right ear while the body writhes in pain. That such painful acts could be a form of healing seems a rather counterintuitive insight. Similarly, when patients in psychiatric institutions repeatedly describe the various side effects of psychotropic medication, it seems counterintuitive for the healer to insist that such severe discomfort is necessary for their recovery.

That which needs to be hurt, pushed aside, or transgressed in order for a person to be healed may well be held dear by the patients. Khalid, a patient in the Clinic for Transcultural Psychiatry at Aarhus University Hospital, told me and his nurse about the long and intimate relation he had with a jinn who called himself Abu Hassan. Abu Hassan would join Khalid in his consultations at the clinic. At one consultation Khalid told his nurse: 'Abu Hassan tells me about you, that you think I'm going to make trouble. He also talks to my friends. He wants me to hate you. He says you want to force me to take medicine, to make me crazy and tired.'

The nurse denied that this was her intention: 'I think it would be an advantage for you to calm down a bit. The medicine might help you protect yourself. But we will not force the tablets down your throat. It's your life. You have to want this yourself [*du skal selv ville det*].'

When at one point the nurse understood that her patient thought the jinn was actually present in her office, she got up from her chair to stand where the jinn was supposed to be. By physically occupying the space of the jinn, she wanted to prove to her patient that the spirit was merely a delusion. He needed to realise the unreality of his inner voice in order to open himself up for proper treatment. Later Khalid explained that the nurse's attempt did not work because Abu Hassan had simply entered her body. Since she was not protected, the jinn could move freely in and out of her body. This was also how it apparently read the nurse's thoughts and passed them on to Khalid.

In the case of Esther and Jørgen's treatment of Aziz, what needed to be pushed aside was not a jinn since Aziz's jinn had already been expelled during exorcisms. Rather it was certain religious thoughts, beliefs, and practices that could be harmful symptoms of psychosis. For Aziz's life to continue, these beliefs had to be restrained or diminished. Thus a certain self-sacrifice was requested of Aziz: namely the sacrifice of that part within him that had submitted itself – perhaps to an unhealthy extent – to what it regarded as divine law.

I think it is hard to imagine how such a self-sacrifice is accomplished. It is neither comparable to a request for suicide, nor to a turning down of the prospect of eternal happiness and boundless pleasure in paradise. To ask a pious self to sacrifice its religious practices may well be like asking it to throw itself directly into the eternal flames of hell. For a person who spends a considerable amount of time meditating upon the turmoil awaiting in the grave – the never-ending suffering and pain, the burning of bones, the smouldering embers under the feet, and the molten brass being poured down the throat to eternally melt away the organs from the inside[3] – it may be difficult to destroy the only chance of avoiding these torments, namely by fulfilling the divine commands.

As described by both Aziz and Abu Samir, and as Abu Bilal frequently confirmed in his weekly lectures at the mosque, 'sleepiness' is what characterises the people of hell. Sleepiness prevents them from obtaining the kind of certitude and faith (*yaqīn*) that comes about only through the fulfilment of religious duties (*'ibādāt*). Only in death will these people wake to see what an eternal nightmare they have prepared for themselves (Quran 67: 6–11). These divine torments are not just abstract and imagined by such pious selves – they may be quite intensely and tangibly tasted in the experience of pain throughout earthly life. The multiple side effects that typically evolve during the onset of psychiatric medication may easily be conceived of as such a forewarning. As Hirschkind (2006: 85) writes in his analysis of Islamic eschatology: 'death [is] made present through regular reflection on the decay of the body, the furrowing of the face, or the death of loved ones. Sensations such as hunger, physical pain, sickness, or the tiring of the muscles after labour [are] also signs, opportunities to recognize the approach to death.'

In contrast to people like Aziz and Abu Samir, for whom psychiatric medication was identified as an outright attack on their souls, I also met several Muslim psychiatric patients who had come to realise that for them psychotropic medicine was a necessary part of their healing. However, they all emphasised how they initially experienced the treatment as rough and transgressive. Most felt as if they had become more ill, as though their existence was being torn apart. It was only later, after realising the necessity of psychotropic drugs and the fact it was an obligation for them to take the medication, that some peace of mind could be obtained. This was the case for an elderly Palestinian woman suffering from depression, whose two adult sons were both being treated for schizophrenia. A middle-aged Moroccan man diagnosed with paranoid schizophrenia had also arrived at this same conclusion. After a number of Islamic treatments, he realised he simply could not combat his jinn without the help of antipsychotic medicine. However, despite the medicine, the voices continued to stay with him along with a number of side effects in the form of shaking and sleepiness, but the voices would be a little less intrusive.

Patients like these often relied on the Quranic statement that, just as God created all illnesses, so He has provided a cure for them all. It is therefore a religious obligation for any ill person to seek the correct cure for their illness (see also Scene 9). Thus they came to realise that what they had tried to defend themselves against was in fact the healing; a misguided attempt to escape the healing of God; and hence they understood the necessity of giving up their defensive reactions against the working of the drugs on their bodies.

That psychiatric medication is not initially experienced as a healing or fortification of the self is not at all surprising considering its significant side effects. The renowned but controversial psychiatrist Peter Breggin (2008) describes how psychotropic drugs effectively work as what he calls 'brain-disabling treatment'. Yet when psychiatrists maintain that psychiatric treatment aims not at the transgression of mental faculties but rather at a fortification of the ego, this derives from an understanding that some emotional fluctuations are dangerous to the self, and even if they are intimately tied to the self, they may usefully be removed or sedated so the self will be strengthened.

What would be strengthened is the capacity of an ego to take its place in modern society as a rationally functioning and self-sustaining individual. This is believed to be not only in the interest of wider society, but also in the interest of the individual. Happiness and 'the good life' within the psychiatric model are perceived as existing in the form of a balanced self-sustainment that comes neither from falling into the depths of paranoia and depression, nor from ascending to hypermania and psychosis. If delusional beliefs or extreme emotional fluctuations are preventing the ego from what is regarded as rational self-sustaining behaviour, these need to be removed, or sacrificed, in order to make the good life possible again.

This conception of the healthy soul is not far from what we find within Islamic traditions of healing. Here emphasis is also placed on establishing a balance and enabling the fulfilment of individual self-interest. Yet the practices and emotional dispositions that best serve individual self-interest are perceived in highly different ways. Pursuing one's self-interest within the Islamic model means pursuing those religious practices that make the 'good life' possible in the hereafter. The fact that religious practices may also result in a good life in this world is not the primary objective.

A further difference is that worship in neo-orthodox Islam has as its primary function the establishing within the individual that it is not possible to sustain one's own life. Hence realisation of total dependence on the divine, rather than self-sustainment, is the ultimate aim within this model of healing. Acknowledgement of such super-dependence is not primarily facilitated through rational scrutiny, but is instead established through emotional arousal. The ability to be emotionally touched by the divine message, to feel and realise it through the 'heart', is of utmost importance. A soul in balance, as perceived in neo-orthodox Islam, is the soul that has established the emotional disposition of gratitude and patience to whatever it faces, alongside equal hope of paradise and fear of hell. To explain what he calls the 'middle way' of Islam, Abu Bilal refers to the Muslim scholar Ibn Qayyim al-Jawziyah's [1292–1350 C.E.] saying that: 'On his way to God, a [believer's] heart is likened to a bird: love is its head, fear and hope are its wings. Hence, when the head and wings are sound, the bird will fly perfectly; if the head is cut, the bird will die and when he loses the wings, he will be inevitably subjected to hunting' (see also Quran 7: 56).

It is in the emphasis on the importance of the emotional faculties of the heart that the Islamic model of healing comes into most direct conflict with the psychiatric one. While psychiatric medication consists primarily of the dampening of irrational delusions and emotions in order to free the brain, the Islamic model aims at the emancipation of the heart. This sometimes means overriding what is regarded as the limited scope of brain intelligence (*'aql*). What needs to be sacrificed in the Islamic treatments is the idea that autonomous and rational control of one's actions is possible; that ultimately one could be master of one's own life.

Despite the different ways in which Islamic and psychiatric treatment tend to emphasise either the cultivation of emotional sensitivity or rational mastery, we should not, however, go so far as to conclude that the idea of individual choice is reserved to the psychiatric system. In fact the possibility of an individual to autonomously choose to obey divine doctrine is highly central to Islamic thought. In much the same way, we can also understand the emphasis on individual autonomy in the psychiatric system as the freedom to obey a particular regime of self-government inherent to secular modernity. While the history of secular modernity is often conceived of as a gradual triumph of individual autonomy, as Asad (2003: 73) points out, we need to consider in more detail the paradox that 'the self to be liberated from external control must be subjected to the control of a liberating self already and always free, aware, and in control of its own desires'.

## Free choice and respectful coercion

If we began this chapter with Csordas's (1987) plea that more attention should be paid to the importance of the sacred in all healing encounters, this discussion of sacrifice as the primary vehicle for acknowledging the sacred may be taking us in different directions. Csordas's emphasis on the construction of sacred and medical realities is reflected in the shift of contemporary theories in medical anthropology to a focus on healing as related to the function of human agency and self-creativity, as in Whyte and Callan's analyses, as well as Taussig's emphasis on the constructed nature of the social fact. If we take the principal object of anthropology to be essentially human in nature, this attention to the creative powers of humans should not come as a surprise. However, as Mattingly (2010) asserts, this has not always been the case.

In rejecting the grand schemes of previously dominant schools such as structuralism and Marxism, anthropologists have for some time attempted to include in their ethnographies a sensitivity for the capacity of human beings to act within the social scene (Barth 1966, 1987; Bourdieu 1977; Ortner 1984; Csordas 1990; Otto and Pedersen 2005). These attempts have centred on concepts such as 'practice', 'embodiment', or 'habitus' that might somehow allow the envisioning of a balanced intertwining of individual choice and social structure. For Mattingly (2010: 51), these attempts have never entirely succeeded. We may encounter individual actors within these frameworks of practice, transaction, or embodiment theory, but in the end their supposedly individual actions still seem to be inevitably caught up by deep social structures. Thus for example Sherry Ortner (1984: 151) points out how most practice theories, despite their attention to the cultural construction of individual interest, often end up emphasising the old economic model of human action and sociality as based on an intrinsic inclination in individuals to accumulate value. Regardless of whether or not it is consciously realised by individual actors, within this model the basic structural driving force of human life is located in economic calculation. According to Mattingly (2010: 52), despite these brave efforts, genuine human agency, moral 'willing', and creativity still escape the anthropological gaze. As Ortner (2006: 2) points out in a critique of structuralist strands in anthropology, we still need to recognise not only how 'history makes people', but also how 'people make history'.

In line with such thinking, Csordas (1997: vii) proposed that in anthropology the answer to the central question of what a human is should start with the investigation of 'how we make ourselves human'. What is central in his thought-provoking account of Catholic charismatic healing is how a healthy and what he calls 'sacred self' comes about, not by the intervention of unseen structural or transcendental forces, but by the efforts of people in defining themselves in terms of the wholly 'other' than human (Csordas 1997: 39). This, to be sure, is a far cry from any neo-liberal fantasy of an autonomous actor. Instead Csordas (1997: 278) aims to show how 'the dualities between preobjective and objective, self and person, or being in the world and representation are not given outside the existential self processes that constitute them'. It is in this subtle sense that charismatic healing can be said to be the result of 'self-creativity'.

How does the preoccupation with human agency and self-creativity in medical anthropology relate to the transgressive, perhaps even sacrificial healing practices we are exploring in Danish psychiatry and Islamic exorcism? Listening to the statements by Jørgen and Esther, it would seem to be working well. In psychiatric healthcare, what needs to be removed in order to be healed are the delusions and unstable emotions that prohibit the 'ego' from acting rationally and controlling its body and mind. 'When it is this that controls you,' as Jørgen explains to Aziz in Scene 4, 'then you don't have your own free will.'

In order for the ego to be free to take control of itself and its body, delusions must be exposed and unstable emotions stabilised. Aziz could not stabilise and control himself by his own force in such a way. As Jørgen points out: 'This is why you were sentenced to treatment, because you couldn't control your own free will.'

Let us pause here, for is this not precisely the paradox of secular modernity described by Asad (2003: 73)? One could say the aim is to stabilise and nurture the individual so that it may become the autonomous creative entrepreneur that appears to be the paradigmatic figure and driving engine of much Western liberal discourse (Mahmood 2005: 7; Hirschkind 2011: 637). Yet, as also pointed out by Mattingly (2010: 52), this notion of an autonomous, responsible individual capable of somehow controlling itself seems deeply rooted in a concept of the human as essentially structured through rational, economic instincts. Illness, in this sense, can be defined as a malfunction of the otherwise ideally rational *homo economicus*. Thus freedom from illness is freedom to submit to an ideal of rational, self-sustaining, economic behaviour. Human agency or 'free will' in this context means succumbing to this economic ideal. Once 'free will' drags the individual towards other ends, then the human capacity for agency becomes a problem to overcome. Then 'free will' needs to be 'controlled', as Jørgen asserts.

By now it should be clear that it is by no means sufficient to talk about a single agency at work within the body of a human. In the context of these practices of healing, it would be better to think of a compound or a multiplicity of agentive forces dragging the body towards various possible destinations. Something within a human can apparently be designated as 'free will', but something else, which constantly threatens to drag free will in undesirable directions, is also present. It is perhaps for this reason that a third element can also be found; namely that observing faculty that is supposed to take control over the 'free will'. The old psychoanalytical distinctions between a lower self or 'id', an 'ego', and a 'super-ego' are to a wide extent upheld, even if not always fully acknowledged, by professionals in Danish psychiatry.[4]

The concept of the self (*nafs*) in Islamic theology is constituted by a comparably complex and ambiguous structure involving both the drives and impulses of bodily desires (*shahawāt*), the intelligence, the capacity of the mind for reasoning (*ʿaql*), and the heart (*qalb*), which, besides directing the circulation of blood, is also the organ that holds the capacity for judgement and for witnessing the truth. Finally, the self comprises a fourth part, often referred to as *rūḥ* (soul), which holds a special connection to and remembrance of the divine. As Pandolfo (2018: 315–19) describes, the 'self' in Islam is the 'enjoiner of evil … the desire for power and possessions, and the passion of anger that causes hatred and violence' but it is also the 'faculty of imagination' (*taṣawwur*), 'the spirit and metaphysical soul'.

In modern usage the term *amrāḍ nafsiyya* (illnesses of the self) is often used to designate psychological illnesses, distinct from *amrāḍ rūḥāniyya* (illnesses of the soul), which by contrast refer to illnesses attributed to a theological domain. However, the majority of Muslims I worked with do not distinguish in this way. Instead they conceive of the *nafs* and the *rūḥ* as both part of an inseparable body–soul complex. In their view, psychological illnesses occur due to a blockage in the circulation because of the influence of *waswās* (devils' whispering) or the intake of harmful substances (see also Philips 2007).[5]

Within the Islamic treatments, force is exercised with the aim of freeing the 'self' to take control of its body and mental processes, but not quite in the same manner as in the psychiatric system. Thus the relevant part of the self that needs to be freed is not so much the mind–brain 'ego', but rather the 'heart' (*qalb*) and its ability to respond emotionally and ethically in accordance with its circumstances (Mahmood 2005; Hirschkind 2006; Pandolfo 2018). What is important is the cultivation of certain virtues so that one may embrace what is being given with gratitude (*shukr*), perseverance, and patience (*ṣabr*) (Sedgwick 2006: 167). The emphasis is not so much on agency in the sense of the ability to act outwardly, as on the ability to receive what is being given with an ethically correct sensitivity.

That which needs to be transgressed is the part of the self occupied with earthly desires, which leads the soul astray from its sole purpose: namely submission to its creator. Frequently the Muslim healer will find that one or more evil jinn are occupying the body of the patient and are taking advantage of a weak self (*al-nafs al-ammāra bil-sū'*) that blindly follows the desires of earthly life. These spirits work to confuse the patient and prevent the soul from submitting itself to the creator. Therefore these spirits need to be cast out or exterminated in order for the soul, through pious worship, to passionately pursue what is recognised as the only source of healing, namely God.

For the jinn, this also involves a sacrifice, since to accept the divine doctrine evoked by the healer inevitably also demands that it leave the body of the possessed. Often its kin or the magician who has sent the jinn will try to kill it for its betrayal. Thus giving up a human body may require a similar leap of faith as that exhibited by Abraham and his son on the mountain of Moriah.

In the case of Nadia who was treated by Abu Bilal (Scene 5), what needed to be transformed was that part of the self which would seek to fulfil its desire with such earthly pleasures as American TV shows or frivolous unrestricted socialising with friends of the opposite sex. Key to the transformation of the self was the removal of the physical manifestation of those desires from her bedroom walls, since these directly prevent angels from entering the room and hence prevent a connection to the divine. Furthermore, what needed to be removed was the idea that she could protect herself against evil simply by hanging a magical image above her bed. This had to be removed in order to facilitate full submission to the only agent that could protect and heal her, namely God. Importantly, Abu Bilal did not remove the images but rather offered the removal of the images as advice to the woman and her father.

As we saw in Chapter 4, the political framework of Danish psychiatric healthcare emphasises above all the importance of actively involving users in all treatment. This is described most clearly in the policy paper outlining the aims and purposes of Aarhus University Hospital at Risskov, which states that psychiatric treatment needs to first and foremost 'take its starting point in the mentally disordered person's own decisions'; that mentally ill persons must be 'treated as equal collaborators with a shared responsibility for reaching the best possible solution'; and that the overall aim of psychiatric intervention is 'to motivate and support the mentally ill to take the greatest possible responsibility for their decisions, self-care, and treatment' (Region Midtjylland 2009: 9–14).

These virtues of individual autonomy are even exercised in situations where, as in the case of Aziz, voluntary commitment to the necessary treatment has proved impossible. With the concept of 'respectful coercion' (*tvang med respekt*), the Ministries of the Interior, Health, and Social Affairs (2005) make it clear how fixation and forced medication can only be applied in situations where the mentally ill have become dangerous either to themselves or to others, and not before all possibilities have been attempted in order to gain the person's voluntary commitment. However, even in such situations, all possible means should continually be applied in order for the patient to voluntarily submit to the treatment. This is why both Jørgen and Esther, in the treatment of Aziz, continue to do their best to explain how important it is he takes the drugs.

The great emphasis on free choice and user involvement expressed in Danish psychiatric healthcare finds a parallel in an often-quoted phrase from Surat al-Baqara (Quran 2: 256) stating 'there shall be no compulsion in religion'. Both Muslim shaykhs and psychiatrists recognise that under special circumstances, the use of force may be necessary if persons have become a threat to themselves or others. Yet in such circumstances, treatment becomes a kind of damage control. To achieve genuine healing, a degree of individual free choice is required. However, it is clear that this choice is often an odd one. Immediately after stating the absence of compulsion in religion, the Quran states: 'The right course has become clear from the wrong. So whoever disbelieves in Taghut and believes in Allah has grasped the most trustworthy handhold with no break in it' (Quran 2: 256).

When the psychiatrist has provided a diagnosis and recommends specific treatment for a given disorder, the right course is made clear in a similar way. In both cases, the choice is between voluntary commitment to treatment and further degrees of pain. Free choice is important, not primarily because people might make better decisions themselves, but because their commitment and acceptance of the treatment is a necessary requirement for its efficacy. Healers and patients might be equals at an abstract level, but in terms of their knowledge of the proper course of action they are not (see also

Ministries of the Interior, Health, and Social Affairs 2005: 11). This is why the role of the psychiatrist is to provide the information or 'psycho-education' needed for the patient to submit to the treatment (see e.g. Aagaard, Merinder, and Mundbjerg 2009).

In both systems, free choice seems to be located in the patients' ability, not to make their own autonomous decisions, but to recognise their powerless situation and accept the right course of action. 'Self-care' in the psychiatric system and in the Islamic forms of healing is about voluntarily accepting the guidance and treatment offered by the healers. Here it is the patients' experience of themselves as independent agents that is sacrificed in favour of allowing the healing agents provided by the healers work upon their bodies. As they do this, their bodies become inscribed into the 'sacred' space of healing. It would be difficult to say the sacralisation occurring at the moment of healing is the result of the patient's own capacity for self-creativity, as Csordas (1997) describes for Catholic charismatic healing. Rather, this particular form of sacralisation lies in their giving up the illusion of any capacity for self-creativity.

While many anthropologists strive to factor a proper concept of human agency into their accounts, healing practices in psychiatric healthcare and Danish mosques seem to be addressing almost the opposite problem, namely how best to control or redirect human agency. Healing and 'emancipation' of the soul in these contexts seem to be centred not so much on a return to human agency as on a subduing of the human capacity to destruct itself. For healing to occur, external, non-human force must be applied to tame and overrule the destructive powers within a human body.

In the last chapter we saw how Jørgen needed to overrule Aziz's conviction that his psychiatric medication was essentially contributing to his illness. Likewise we have seen how Abu Bilal played down Feisal's understanding of the problem in his leg as the abode of the jinn. While Abu Bilal stated with full conviction that Feisal was in fact suffering from the attacks of jinn, Feisal's own experience of these attacks as coming from his lower leg was overruled as a 'psychological problem'. The attempt by Nadia and her father to achieve a form of protection from malevolent beings by hanging an image above her bed was thoroughly transgressed as in fact being a vehicle of the illness. Such transgressive, sacrificial moments seem to be of prime importance in these healing practices. If there is a single twist to the practices of shaykhs, nurses, and psychiatrists that has continued to provoke my analysis, it is this. The next chapter examines how such sacrifices of healing are facilitated by the disruption of individual agency and perception through the evocation of an infinitely larger world of vision, which I propose can be encapsulated with Merleau-Ponty's concept of the 'view from everywhere' and Deleuze's concept of the 'time-image'.

## Notes

1 For a discussion of the various meanings and practices of veiling and unveiling see Saba Mahmood (2005: 23, 50ff), Mayanthi Fernando (2010, 2014), Nadia Fadil (2011), and Karen Waltorp (2018).

2 Most Muslim theologians agree that the son in this story was Ismael and not Isaac as stated in the Bible (Genesis 22). Ismael and his mother Hajar were sent away because of the envy of Abraham's first wife Sarah who, after Ismael was born, miraculously gave birth to Isaac at an old age. According to hadith, Hajar accepted being sent away as a command of God. Left alone with her son in the desert of Faras – the area now called Mecca – Hajar desperately searched for water. After running seven times up and down the hills of al-Safa and al-Marwa, Ismael's heel struck a stone, which revealed the miraculous well of Zamzam. The water saved Hajar and Ismael. Today Muslims use water from the Zamzam well for a wide variety of healing purposes, including the expelling of jinn during exorcisms. In Islamic theology, Abraham's ascent to the summit of Moriah thus initiates a chain of sacrifices – most importantly the self-sacrifice of Ismael and his mother, which is also commemorated during the obligatory pilgrimage to Mecca (*ḥajj*).

3 These are some of the torments I heard about during my fieldwork. The classic meditation on the topic is Al-Ghazali's (1989) *Remembrance of Death*. For a vivid exposition, some of the young people I worked with recommended Anwar Al-Awlaki's (2010) controversial description of 'Hellfire'.

4 Jørgen Aagaard explains how current rejections of psychoanalysis are a result of the failure of psychoanalytic therapy to produce evidence of any measurable effect. Yet for him, the theoretical framework of psychoanalysis still provides the main tools for understanding the human psyche. In this he frequently refers to the Danish psychiatrist Erling Jacobsen's (1984) work on the foundational processes of the mind (see also Freud 2003: 119. See Luhrmann 2000 for an analysis of the dynamics between psychotherapy and biomedical psychiatry in the US).

5 Philips (2007: 10ff) describes the differences in opinion among Muslim scholars regarding the *nafs* and *rūḥ*, some arguing that the two terms can be used interchangeably, others arguing that they refer to essentially different entities in the constitution of human consciousness.

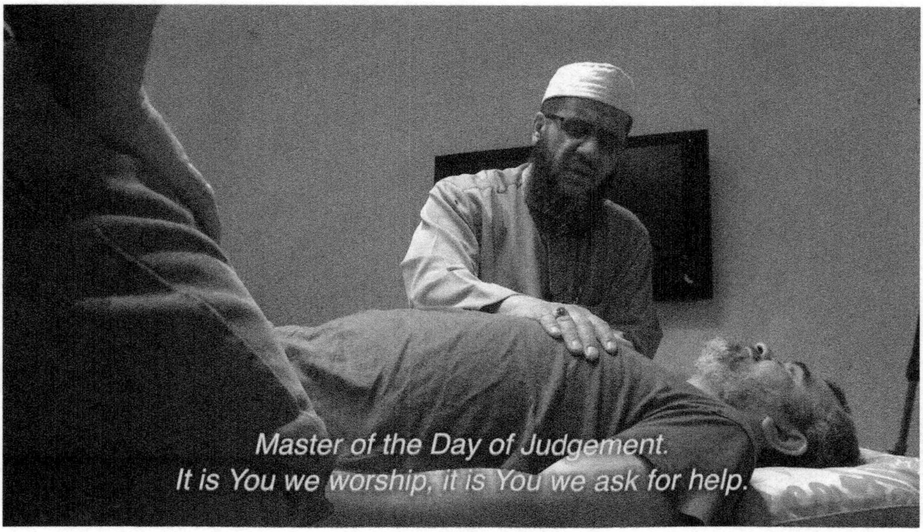
Master of the Day of Judgement.
It is You we worship, it is You we ask for help.

6.1 Still from Scene 2

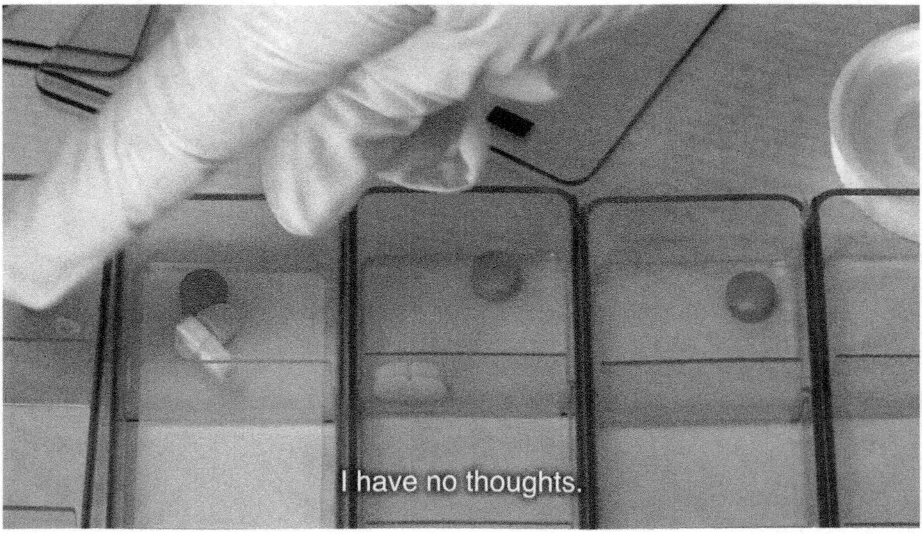
I have no thoughts.

6.2 Still from Scene 8

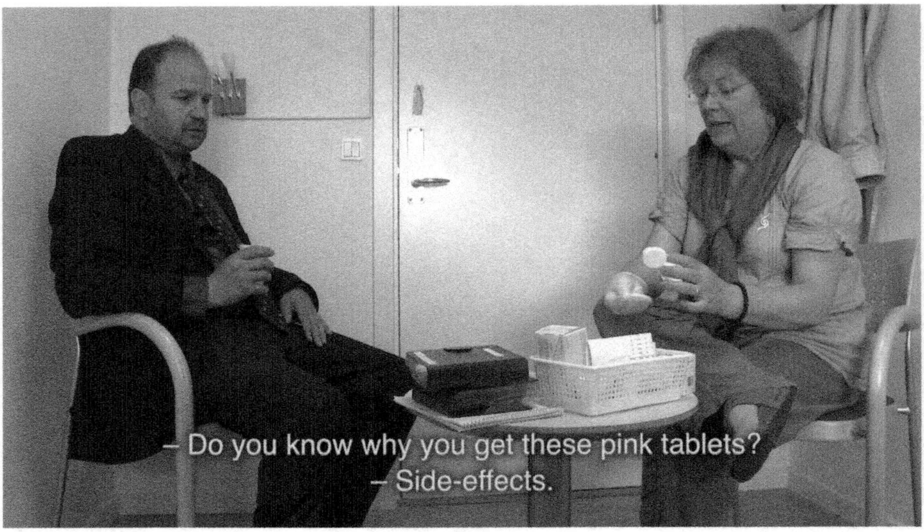
– Do you know why you get these pink tablets?
– Side-effects.

6.3 Still from Scene 8

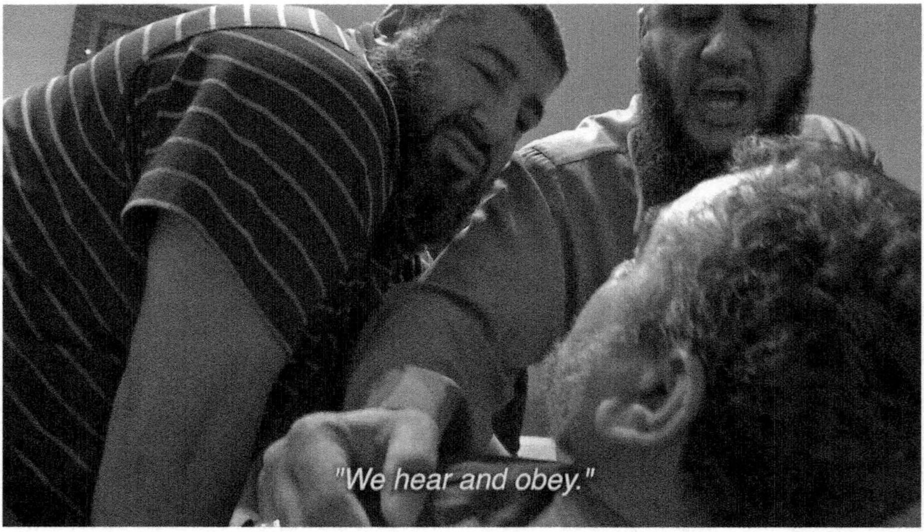
"We hear and obey."

6.4 Still from Scene 2

6

# *Ruqya*, psychotropics, and montage

In May 2011, Abu Omar, a highly devoted and practising member of the Society for Equality and Brotherhood in Brabrand, was found sitting on the floor of the mosque as though his soul had completely departed this world. It happened in much the same way as when Feisal had first gone into the state of *ṣarʿ* nine months before. In the last section of the evening prayer (*ṣalāt al-ʿishāʾ*) Abu Omar kept kneeling, refusing to bow during the obligatory prostrations, in which the forehead touches the ground. According to the people I worked with, this is the situation where the believer reaches the closest proximity to the divine – a moment of staring right into the unseen face of God. I was standing a few metres to the right of Abu Omar, but had not noticed he was merely sitting in the latter part of the prayer.

When the prayer is finished, Abu Bilal walks straight towards him. He says something, but Abu Omar just slides backwards onto the floor. His eyes are empty, staring towards the ceiling. The men in the mosque quickly gather around him and try to wake him up; they measure his pulse, offer him water. Abu Omar's five-year-old son walks around nervous, confused, looks at his father. Someone tries to comfort him and takes him out of the room.

Abu Bilal sits down next to Abu Omar and tries to call him back to life, but nothing happens. There are only these empty eyes, frozen to an imperceptible point on the ceiling. I worry about whether this is a kind of thrombosis or stroke, but when I ask Erdam if an ambulance should be called, he says he doesn't think so. Abu Bilal starts to recite Surat al-Fatiha – the opening verse of the Quran – with his right hand pressed close to Abu Omar's chest, just above the heart. Abu Bilal reads for a long time, repeating the verse over and over. Abu Muhammad holds Abu Omar's left arm and measures his pulse with his fingers. For the first time I see Abu Muhammad worried; this huge man, usually calm as a rock.

Nothing happens. I just sit here next to Abu Omar, feeling more and more uneasy. His face is pale and devoid of life. The lips and nostrils are still, but a slight movement of his chest reveals that he is breathing. Abu Bilal continues to recite and many minutes pass like this. Then suddenly Abu Omar's right index finger stretches out. The muscles in his thighs and stomach appear to contract. He bends upwards. His face turns reddish, the teeth and left fist tightly clenched. He moves towards Abu Bilal, and looks as though he wants to hit him. The men push him back. I join in and help with pushing – somehow relieved I can do something.

'Who are you?' Abu Bilal cries.

The blood seems to rush to Abu Omar's head. He wheezes something completely incomprehensible. His voice is husky. His eyes are slits. He tries to bend up again but we keep him down and Abu Bilal continues to recite. The guttural voice returns. It is in the Iraqi dialect and I do not understand any of it. Later I am told that he cried: 'What do you want?' and 'You're not a shaykh, you're a woman.'

Abu Bilal raises his voice, shouts to the jinn that if it does not exit, he will continue to recite until the morning prayer. He demands it exits from the toe. This is important, since a jinn exiting from a person's head might cause serious brain damage. Abu Bilal points downwards towards the feet: 'Get out.'

Abu Omar's face is soaked in sweat, the stomach swollen and deformed, and his feet move quickly from side to side. Everything else in the body is kept tightly to the floor by all of us. Abu Bilal demands the *shahāda*: 'Testify that there's no god but God and that Muhammad is his prophet.'

A man comes in with a glass of water. He wants to sprinkle it on Abu Omar but instead it hits all of the men holding the head, arms, and legs of the possessed.

'Stop it,' Abu Bilal shouts, 'what is the reason for this water?'

The man stops immediately and walks out. Abu Bilal continues the reading. The veins at Abu Omar's throat and temples are bulging. I hope these guys know what they're doing. I hope I know what I'm taking part in. Please God, heal this man.

We are looking at him from all sides. Every gesture of this body receives a reaction. Yet taking part in this panoptic gaze I feel nothing but uncertainty. Is there something here that still escapes our attention? His pulse, the resurfacing of traumatic memories from the war in Iraq, or utterances that are so difficult to understand that not even his Iraqi friends can comprehend them? What if he is trying to tell Abu Bilal that he needs a doctor? Abu Bilal recites even louder.

Then finally something happens. Something is relaxed and weeping comes in long staggered breaths. The voice has changed: 'Shaykh, shaykh,' it stammers slowly. It is Abu Omar again. He is exhausted; his voice is weak. I think he asks where he is. Abu Bilal stops the recitation and explains what happened, asks what Abu Omar remembers. He remembers that he was praying, but except for that, nothing. He looks drained and despondent. He is lifted up so that he can sit. The veins have relaxed again and his skin is turning pale.

The men in the mosque appear disturbed. His friend Erdam asks several times: 'How – a person who prays and fasts – how can this be?' Erdam has told me many times how psychological and jinn-related illnesses never hit a true believer since they are caused by disobedience to God. But Abu Omar is clearly not disobedient. His actions testify to his virtues. He prays and fasts, he performs all of the obligatory ablutions and nearly all of the voluntary prayers. Erdam is shocked; how could this happen to such a man?

But Abu Bilal says that the first time he met Abu Omar last year, he felt something was not right, that he needed treatment with *ruqya*. Tonight it finally broke out. Abu Bilal recites over a glass of water that Abu Omar drinks. Now he is able to stand. He leaves the prayer room to do the ritual ablutions in order to repeat the obligatory evening prayer he just missed. I talk to Bilal, the son of the shaykh and a few of the other young guys who witnessed the scene.

'I think it was a jinn,' Bilal says, 'but there wasn't any blood. Often there's blood on the big or little toe if the jinn exits. But not always.'

Bilal thinks the jinn left when the weeping started. The men in the mosque joke about the jinn, that it is now sitting over there on that chair, pointing at Abu Mustafa, the chief of the small cafe next to the mosque. Abu Bilal makes fun of the guy who wanted to exorcise the jinn by sprinkling water on all of us.

I don't know what to think when I drive home this evening. I think I need a cigarette. I think I shouldn't smoke, that it's not wise now. What type of analysis should I make? I could connect the fact that Abu Bilal had, just before the whole thing happened, given a lecture about *ruqya sharʿiyya*. He explained in detail about the jinn, how one should not be afraid of them as one should only be afraid of God. Then suddenly this happens to one of the most faithful in the mosque. What does this tell us? Did Abu Omar need this form of attention or emotional outlet? Does something within him need to hit Abu Bilal and cry? And if it really is an alien spirit, what kind of analysis do I then produce? Then this is just the way it is. A description. An account of something to which I can add nothing more. Only God knows.

I stop the car, get out and light the cigarette. I am standing beside the rubbish bins close to my home. I walk away from them. A light drizzle hits my face. I ask for God's protection, then ask if God really exists. I try to force the sneaking doubt away, the devils' whispering. I ask for forgiveness. I inhale the smoke. Nothing in my mind seems to fit together. I feel my legs shake; dizziness. I walk to my house and when I enter, I lock the door from the inside. The evil jinn leave a house if you greet them with God's peace (*salāmu ʿalaykum*) when entering. I am inside this house with all the pictures on the walls, alcohol in the cupboards – here in this house where the jinn can rule as freely as they want. I hope nothing has followed me on the way home from the mosque. I know I shouldn't be afraid of the jinn. As I start to write this fieldnote my left index finger begins to vibrate. I know this feeling from before, but I don't like that it starts now.

It stops. Thank you, God.

## Cinema fist

I have suggested the term self-sacrifice as somehow useful in understanding healing in psychiatric healthcare and Islamic exorcism, but I have not specifically discussed how such sacrifices may be performed in healing. So far in this account I have discussed how healers and patients move between different states of doubt, resignation, certainty, and faith. Through the oscillation between these states, a situation or condition of mind is established in which the submission of the self to an all-powerful invisible truth becomes possible. But what perceivable form does this externality take in the healing encounter? How is the invisible made present? What kind of mediation allows it to succeed in subjugating the patient to its force? What role does the nurse, the psychiatrist, or the shaykh play as mediums of this power?

This chapter brings the concept of montage – as proposed in Eisenstein's, Vertov's, and Deleuze's theories of cinema – into play alongside Kierkegaard's double movement of faith and Merleau-Ponty's notion of the invisible as an infinitely vast, ever-present, yet unreachable 'view from everywhere' (Merleau-Ponty 1964: 51; 2002: 79; Kelly 2005; Holbraad and Willerslev 2007). Merleau-Ponty argues that while inaccessible to us, this totality of vision underlies and provides the necessary ground for any particular situated perspective. Indeed it is the precondition for our possibility of perceiving anything. This ultimate anonymous viewpoint – which could only ever be taken up by a divine being – was arguably what the early Soviet filmmakers attempted to tap into by way of cinematic montage (Eisenstein 1928; Vertov 1929, 1984: 15–17). Indeed, they tried to immerse themselves in this impossible viewpoint to the extent that they could use montage as a 'cinema fist' to change and reconstruct the entire constitution of their world (Eisenstein 1988: 64). Here I use this figure of montage as a so-called 'cinema fist' in analysing the work of the nurse, the psychiatrist, and the shaykh who in the act of healing, as knights of faith, must in a comparable way take on the obligation of becoming seers, knowers, and masters of the invisible powers inflicting their patients' pain (see also Suhr 2017).

Not only must the healers see and know. They must also take on the task of hurting, transgressing, converting, or exterminating that within the patient which is inflicting the pain. I suggest that the overpowering of that which is causing the pain, however differently this might be conceived of within the two healing systems, is accomplished by the insertion of a compound object of extraordinary knowledge and power into the body of the patient. With Merleau-Ponty we may conceptualise this tremendous object faced by the patients during the act of healing as an object containing nothing less than the panoptic 'view from everywhere'. Confronted with the paradoxical and impossible 'view from everywhere', that will which hurts within the patient can do nothing but subject itself to it. The small psychotropic tablet and the evidence-based aura of the vast realm of biomedicine that it is invested with can be understood in this way. Despite its minute size, it is served to the patient as a distillate in tablet form of truly universal power and knowledge.

Within neo-orthodox Islam, Merleau-Ponty's concept of an all-pervading perception from all places and all times is evoked through three of the ninety-nine-plus names for God, the All-Seeing (*al-Baṣīr*), the All-Hearing (*al-Samī'*), and the All-Knowing (*al-'Alīm*). The Quran as recited and blown by the healer with short sharp breaths into the right ear of the possessed – the Quran as a substrate of such omnipresent perception, a form of ultimate montage (Hirschkind 2006: 155; Khan 2009) – is, like the tablet, introduced into the possessed in order to explode and overpower the alien agency at work in their body. Thus the possessed body in the moment of healing becomes the battleground not only of healer and illness, but also of Abraham, Moses, Solomon, Muhammad, and numerous additional prophets, jinn, and *shayāṭīn* through the recitation of multiple fragments of verses from the Quran. The number of agentive powers radically multiplies through the recitation, but in such a way that all fragments and perspectives are reorganised and surrendered to the one divine being holding the power over it all.

Within this very healing moment lies the ever-present danger of heresy, of conflating the agency the healer has borrowed from the invisible with her or his own agency. If the invisible is indeed invisible, no human being can see what it encompasses. Yet I wonder whether all of us holding this struggling body are not in fact, from the point of view of Abu Omar's jinn, representing exactly that panoptic 'view from everywhere' that Merleau-Ponty describes in his theory of perception. At this moment of healing we stand in for the whole, the community, God's umma, to which Abu Omar and his jinn need to reattach. The agencies battling each other for ownership of the besieged body have become separate from the truth and unity of God. Yet on closer inspection, our actualisation of the whole is also incomplete and detached from the 'holy'. As Marion (2002: 150–7) points out, all actualisations of the holy must necessarily be incomplete, since it is only as an absence that the holy can be approached in actual experience (see also Steinbock 2007; Willerslev and Pedersen 2010).

For me at least, being part of this panoptic viewpoint that weaves itself from all sides through the body of Abu Omar is to experience not unity, but separation. When I look at the worried gazes of Abu Muhammad and

Erdam, I feel that at this moment we share not a unification with God, but another degree of distance.

I try to imagine what Abu Bilal is experiencing in this moment. In his recitation of multiple Quranic fragments, Abu Bilal speaks directly with the voice of God, the voices of the prophets, even the voices of the jinn. In this way he embodies the closest proximity to the ultimate viewpoint. Yet he has often explained to me how, every time he conducts a sermon or Quranic healing, he says a special prayer to remind himself that it is also he who needs these recitations.

As Pandolfo (1997: 241) points out, the work of a healer involves standing on the edge between the visible and the invisible. Tapping into the invisible and using the 'cinema fist' of the Creator carries the risk of venturing astray into the idolatrous thought that by one's own power, one could be 'self-creative' (Sedgwick 2006: 56; Steinbock 2007: 212). While developed in a Catholic context, Marion's (2002) theory that the experience of God is always and necessarily predicated on absence and distance seems to hold true here. The more Abu Bilal comes to embody the holy, the more he needs to distance and humble himself.

Humanism – or, more precisely, belief in the human capacity to overcome obstacles of social life through dialectical reasoning – was also the object of Deleuze's criticism of the montage school of the early Soviet filmmakers. These filmmakers identified in cinema the key tools for moving humankind through the so-called Marxist–Hegelian dialectic of thesis–antithesis towards synthesis.[1] For them, montage was a way of visibly exposing the illnesses of capitalist society and designating the cures needed for the establishment of communist utopia.

In criticising Eisenstein's dialectical montage, Deleuze (2005b: 203) proposed an alternative philosophy of film. Key to his theorisation of film is the idea that 'human creativity' begins by recognising the essential powerlessness and incapacity of subjective human thought. Despite Deleuze's frequent rejections of religion, there seems to be something rather 'religious', 'mystical', perhaps even 'Islamic' about his mode of thinking (Lovat and Semetsky 2009). In a comparison of Deleuzian film theory with Islamic art, Marks (2010: 18) points out how both Deleuze's cinema theory and much Islamic theology emphasise the necessity of a suspension of our perceived capacity for action and judgement. As Marks (2010: 17) observes, both the Islamic concept of *fanā'* – described in Sufism and mainstream Sunni theology as a state of total annihilation of the self in remembrance of God – and Deleuze's concept of creativity involve the idea that the 'psychic organization that both allows us to survive and prevents us from really being alive has to be (gently) taken apart'. Deleuze identified modern cinema as the medium that could best facilitate such a dismantling of normal subject-centred perception. As he writes (2005b: 161): 'What cinema advances is not the power of thought but its "impower" … the impossibility of thinking that is thought.'

Deleuze detects a profound break occurring in the evolution of cinema between a movement-image and a time-image. With the movement-image he identifies types of cinema that – as with Eisenstein or as in Hollywood continuity editing – subordinate time to movement in space (Deleuze 2005a[1986]: 30ff). The movement-image constitutes an indirect image of time, because time flows from human action and re-action. The movement-image evokes history as a progression of linear or spiral events that take place as a consequence of the dialectics between humans and their environment.

According to Deleuze, the movement-image of classical cinema – and the trust it showed in the capacity of human agency and reasoning – suffered a huge disturbance in the mid-twentieth century. Awakening to the devastating disasters of the Second World War, humankind found itself in a situation where it was no longer possible to see history as progress. As Deleuze (2005b: 166) points out, the world looked like a bad film, a movement-image in reverse: 'The modern fact is that we no longer believe in this world.'

This situation gave rise to a new type of cinema that aimed not to imitate action (as in Hollywood) or create the condition for human action (as in Eisenstein or Vertov), but to show human action as a function of time – a differentiation of time unfolding from inside time itself. The time-image of modern cinema is thus the suspension of the dialectic. Rather than providing spectators with the narrative tools or scripts to make history and become actors, the time-image creates the condition for 'seeing', rendering the viewer into a 'seer' or a 'witness' observing the situation of humankind from a point outside of human subjective thought, vision, and action. As Deleuze (2005b: 163) writes: 'the cinematographic image, as soon as it takes on its aberration of movement, carries out a *suspension of the world* or affects the visible with a *disturbance*, which, far from making thought visible, as Eisenstein wanted, are on the contrary directed to what does not let itself be thought in thought, and equally to what does not let itself be seen in vision.'

For Deleuze, the seer – whose visionary experiences exceed what can actually be seen, thought, or reacted to – has a special ability to accept circumstances, even ones as harsh as those of the Second World War. From the point of view of the seer, '[t]he intolerable is no longer a serious injustice, but the permanent state of a daily banality' (2005b: 164). According to Deleuze, the time-image does not document the world, but reinstates the possibility of belief in this world; that this world is possible through a leap into faith. Referring to Kierkegaard, Deleuze points out how film 'sends us back to an absolute relation with the outside, beyond the inward psychological consciousness, but equally beyond the relative external world, and finds that it alone is capable of restoring the world and the ego to us' (2005b: 171). Unlike Eisenstein's 'cinema fist', which aimed to provide the masses with the conceptual weapons to overthrow their oppressors, Deleuze posits a different 'cinema fist' that evolves through various mechanisms of montage, which also aim to shock the viewer into a revelation of an emancipatory nature, but with a shock that above all underlines the inadequacy of human thought and action.

These cryptic formulations resemble in several ways my Muslim interlocutors' understanding of divine creativity and the healing potential of submitting one's faith to it (*tawakkul ʿalā Allāh*). As Abu Bilal explained quite simply during an evening class in the mosque: 'If I understand that everything I do and everything that happens to me is not in my hands then I don't need to feel misery when experiencing misfortune. I understand that it is good and accept it.' Precisely this act of giving oneself up to the workings of an externality beyond the reach of the human subject is the principal target of the Islamic practices of *ruqya*.

Marks's (2010) comparison of Islamic and New Media Art exposes how Deleuzian theory departs from Islamic mysticism in its insistence on what she calls 'immanent infinity'; the idea of an infinity that cannot be reduced to any singular unity, but is constantly in the process of pluralising. While Islam ultimately locates the infinite and the invisible in a transcendental God as the all-powerful origin and endpoint of everything, Deleuze operates in an open system where the infinite 'cannot contract down to a One' (Marks 2010: 20). Rather, the universe unfolds infinitely, with time as the constant drive forward. In the Deleuzian model, as Marks observes, '[t]hings can't fold back up to where they came from'. In the next chapter we will discuss how this difference between immanent and transcendental infinity has important consequences for the ways in which freedom and agency can be understood. Yet, as Marks (2010: 12) argues, we should not overemphasise these differences. Since God, the all-powerful deity of Islam, is invisible and infinitely beyond our grasp, any human quest for unity with God will always remain incomplete. The quest of getting close to God involves giving oneself up to a whole, which, since it cannot be fully contemplated, will necessarily remain open. For our purposes we observe here the parallel to Merleau-Ponty's (2002) understanding of the 'perceptual faith' involved at the level of our tiniest motor-intentional actions, such as gripping coffee cups (see Chapter 1).

In an analysis of anti-sorcery rituals in Sri Lanka, Bruce Kapferer (2013) points out how ritual always had the 'cinematic' qualities we now find in modern cinema. Like Marks in her analysis of the links between medieval Islamic art and modern media art, Kapferer inverts the evolution of modern cinema by pointing out how archaic rituals anticipate the potential of cinematic montage by confronting ritual participants with multiple and contradictory viewpoints. As he states: 'aside from the obvious differences of cinema and ritual there is an underlying unity' (2013: 21; 2014; see also Behrend, Dreschke, and Zillinger 2015). Kapferer shows that cinema as an analytical model of ritual allows for a different view of the transformative potential of ritual; one that has been downplayed in customary interpretations of ritual as drama or theatre. Ritual, Kapferer argues, is not, as many anthropologists have suggested, primarily about subject-centred embodiment and the symbolic performance of mythology. Like cinema, ritual is a continuous emerging, shaping, and reshaping of subject-positioning that works to collapse any sense of singular bodily unity. Like a Deleuzian montage machine, ritual works by exploding the perspectives of the ritual participants, thereby allowing renewed access to the realm of the 'virtual'. As also pointed out by Marks (2010: 14), Deleuze's notion of virtuality as an imperceptible field of possibility from which actual existence arises lies close to Islamic descriptions of the creative powers of God.

In this chapter I consider the Islamic treatments and the consultations in Danish psychiatry as spaces for the performance of this kind of ritual. The form of dissolution achieved by these rituals bears a resemblance to Victor Turner's (1967: 95) classic description of the 'liminal' inversion of everyday life that marks the threshold between a person's 'pre-ritual status' and the status the person is supposed to obtain after ritual. Yet the rituals I describe here are not intended to bring about a return to the state of everyday affairs. For the patients entering into these ritual spaces, the everyday, like the past, is that which needs to be left behind. The ritual is intended as part of a total transformation in which the patient as well as the healer is absorbed within the space of the liminal (see also Mahmood 2005: 131).

In the Islamic case it is obviously God who is understood as the transformative agent. In Danish psychiatry the patients need not submit themselves to God, but instead to the workings of biomedicine, which, however, shares certain characteristics with the divinity worshipped in the mosques. Let us consider more closely how such a ritual montage machine could be at work both in Danish psychiatry and in Islamic exorcisms of jinn. In the following passages we will start with a discussion of the medication given to Aziz in Scene 8 and then move to discuss the exorcism of Abu Omar featured in Scene 2.

## Zyprexa

When reading the prescription insert of the antipsychotic medication given to Aziz in Scene 8, one quickly finds oneself in the unsettling land of montage. Zyprexa (a registered trademark of the pharmaceutical company

Eli Lilly), that unremarkable little white pill, at first glance looks innocent and could easily be overlooked, but once we enter the world of knowledge hiding within it, we are in the abyss. Made from olanzapine, Zyprexa is used in the treatment of illnesses ranging from schizophrenia and other types of psychosis to obsessive compulsive disorder, bipolar disorder, and depression. A wide variety of effects can result from the exposure of the human brain to olanzapine. Reported side effects include restlessness, weight gain, breast milk production, breast development in men, sleepiness, insomnia, constipation, urinary retention, dry mouth, irritability, impaired judgement, swallowing problems, discoloration of teeth, problems keeping body temperature regulated, missed periods, apathy and lack of emotional response, diabetes, brain zaps, auditory hallucinations, runny nose, irreversible movement disorder (tardive dyskinesia), and the rare but life-threatening neuroleptic malignant syndrome.[2]

Multiple chemical agents are set in motion and rearranged when a patient begins to take Zyprexa, but Aziz, however, is prescribed not only Zyprexa but also simvastatin (to control elevated cholesterol) and orphenadrine (to reduce muscle spasms; Danish brand name Lysantin). While the effects of olanzapine in combination with simvastatin and orphenadrine have been studied, the ways in which all these drugs work on patients of Palestinian or Lebanese origin are not fully documented. Since most studies of psychotropics are carried out in Northern Europe or North America, it is often unclear how precisely they work on the bodies and brains of people from other parts of the world. Indeed the psychotropic cocktail consumed by many of these patients is a true experiment in human and biochemical montage. The nurses I worked with repeatedly complained that their non-Danish patients reported symptoms that were not at all covered in the otherwise extensive lists of side effects.

Not only do the drugs in themselves contain a complex montage of chemical agents, but their interaction with the human body in conjunction with other psychotropics produces assemblages of even greater complexity. The effects of these constellations are to some extent reported in the often voluminous patient records. These files include records of each and every meeting between the patient and all the physicians, nurses, social workers, psychiatrists, and psychologists who have been involved in their treatment. Each health professional reports their analysis of the problems and suffering of the patient, proposes their best recommendations for treatment, and reiterates the patient's own account. For the untrained eye it is difficult reading. I quickly felt trapped and lost in the multitude of voices, chemical agents, and symptoms.

When I met Aziz in 2011, the four volumes of his records covered more than twenty years, sixteen hospitalisations, and hundreds of consultations. For the nurse and the psychiatrist who have learned to read these files, they offer glimpses into the suffering of the patient they are dealing with – 'views from everywhere and every then'. Yet it can only be partial and momentary glimpses, as the accumulated files are often too massive and too incomprehensible to be contained within the limits of a single person's memory. This vast and continuously evolving body of knowledge represented by the patient records, the drugs, the trials, and the research literature on the drugs constitutes the invisible ground on which psychiatric treatment takes place. The small psychotropic tablet condenses all of this into a single figure, a particular kind of 'time-image', that answers to the patient's past and present and designates the possibilities of the future. Nothing prevents the patient from accessing the enormous body of knowledge that lies encapsulated within the psychotropic tablet, but for the limits of human memory and comprehension that are simply not equipped to contain it.

Considering the complexity of most psychotropics, it is not hard to imagine how embarking on treatment with a drug such as Zyprexa entails a significant leap of faith. As stated clearly on the declaration, these drugs not only have the power to heal, they can also harm and even kill.

These antipsychotic tablets may relieve the patient from psychosis, but under certain circumstances they could inflict additional psychotic delusions. In the case of olanzapine, McGlashan et al. (2006: 790) conclude – on the basis of a one-year randomised double-blind trial against a placebo – that a significant beneficial treatment effect for psychosis could not be demonstrated. Yet McGlashan et al. also conclude that nearly significant treatment differences suggest that olanzapine might delay the onset of psychosis. Healy (2006) comes to a more disturbing conclusion. In a survey of a large number of FDA trials he claims that adverse effects of olanzapine have effectively resulted in 'the highest rate of suicides in psychotropic trial history' (Healy 2006: 76).[3] As discussed in Chapter 4, similar findings have been published about antidepressants. They may relieve the patient from a state of depression, but they may also burden the patient with even deeper degrees of depression (see for a discussion Parker, Anderson, and Haddad 2003; Bloom 2010; Kirsch 2010).

The power of psychotherapeutic medicine is akin not to the compassionate, ever-forgiving Man-God of the New Testament, but to the divinity of the Old Testament or the Quran: a divinity who might heal, but at other times might severely hurt its subjects. These medicines do not simply protect life, as suggested by the Foucauldian concept of bio-power, but combine aspects of pastoral power (see Chapter 4) with the threatening potential of sovereign power (Foucault 1982; 1988: 278).

To embark upon treatment with Zyprexa, patients need to lay aside their doubts and fears about harm, and offer themselves up to the workings of the drug. Rather than reassuming human agency, patients need to become witnesses to and testimonies of the biochemical agencies at work in their bodies. As a ritual event, psychiatric consultations may be understood as the exposure of the psychosis and the human subject to the vastness of biomedical knowledge. Like the direct image of time described by Deleuze, this body of knowledge crosscuts through space and time, revealing itself as a point of origin through which past, present, and future unfold and come into being. In the healing encounter, this knowledge works by absorbing the patients' personal trajectories of fortune and misfortune into the logical, yet ultimately uncontainable workings of the psychopharmacological universe. For the healer, however, it is not always an easy task to invite their patients along with them into the world of psychotropic medication. Often they meet significant resistance, and their efforts do not always succeed.

## A nice tie

Aziz and Esther's relationship goes back several years. Their weekly conversations seem to me to be repetitions of repetitions, as if they were rehearsing a script. They appear to have a good relationship, and seem to like and respect each other for the part they need to play in the script. The accounts of Aziz's life and problems, his psychotic episodes, and hospitalisations are reiterated each Monday, with small variations. First the greeting, the talk about the general state of things, then the discussion about whether or not Aziz is taking his medicine, whether he is doing his exercises in the gym, if he has been angry at anyone, then the handing over of the blue box containing the weekly dose of psychotropics, finally the weighing, and then the goodbye.

I had followed and recorded the consultations for a while. One day in April 2011 when Esther was particularly busy, their interaction was intensified in a way that made me think about how the aesthetics of montage could be used as an analytics to understand the submission of self facilitated in the psychiatric institutions:

'How are you, Aziz?' Esther begins.

'I'm fine.' This is Aziz's standard answer every Monday.

'You're fine.' Esther is not completely convinced.

'Nice and easy.'

Aziz smiles at Esther. They have had this exchange many times before. Esther is on a tight schedule today so she decides to skip further enquiry into Aziz's present condition.

'Your blood tests have come back. I can see you have taken at least some of the medicine.'

'I have taken it all.'

'You take it all, then that's good. It's in the normal range, so I believe it.'

Esther starts to insert the many tablets into the small compartments of the blue pill box. She notices the resistance in Aziz's answers to her questions. She decides to remind him that what she is doing here really is for his own benefit: 'It's because we care for you, Aziz. We want you to be well. This is what we want.'

'I'm well.' Aziz seems slightly annoyed that he has to confirm his good condition once again.

Esther decides to use the situation to rehearse the effects of the different pills with Aziz.

'Now when I sort out the medicine I can ask if you know why you have to take it. Do you know why you get these pink tablets?'

'Side effects.'

'Do you have any side effects?'

'No.'

'But you get these for the side effects. What about your thoughts – how are they?'

'I have no thoughts.'

'You must have some? This thinking about people you could be angry with, don't you do this?' Esther is still searching for a way into Aziz's interior condition. A recognition of a problem. Denial of problems is part of Aziz's psychotic behaviour.

'No, thank you. I'm not angry with anyone, I like everyone.' Aziz has rehearsed the answers to Esther's questions many times. I am not sure to what extent Aziz is aware that his positive answers might be interpreted as signs of positive psychotic symptoms. But then negative answers to these questions could also be interpreted as signs of an upcoming psychotic episode. Instead by answering Esther's question politely but with this constant twist of irony, he seems to have the upper hand in the discussion.

'Do people like you too? Do they want to talk to you?'

'Yes, all of them talk to me. I'm a nice person.'

Esther decides to drop the topic and enquires into Aziz's knowledge about the other tablets. 'These brown ones – do you know why you get these?'

'No. [Pause.] For the blood?'

'Yes, because there's too much fat in your blood.'

'But it's better now, right?'

'It will be better, because it reduces the amount of fat in your blood. Do you also think about it when eating?'

'I go to the fitness centre.'

'This is good, but you can also consider it when eating. Do you eat a lot of cakes?'

'Three times a week.'

'All these things with fat are not good for you.'

At this point in the conversation Esther appears to regain territory. Aziz exposed himself by pointing out how he exercises in the gym. This answer was not protected by irony and thus Esther suddenly has a hook into her patient. She acknowledges Aziz's efforts in the gym but points out how this is not enough and how he also needs to reduce his fat intake.

'What about the white tablets, Zyprexa – why do you get these?'

'I don't know.' Aziz knows quite well why he has to take these tablets. His answer reveals his resistance to the treatment and how he believes the antipsychotics are in fact harming him.

'Why is it that you need them?'

'Yes, it's Zyprexa.'

'What do they do in the body?'

'What do you mean?'

'How do they work on you?'

'They make you calm.'

'Then it's easier for you to sleep, right?'

'Yes, I sleep well, like a stone. I sleep at ten and wake up at ten.'

'Zyprexa also makes you psychologically stronger. That's why it's important that you take all of it. Here's for a week.' Esther hands Aziz the blue box of pills.

'Thanks for the dinner.'

'Do you want this to carry it?' Esther offers Aziz a small plastic bag.

'It doesn't matter. Is this a nice tie?' Aziz lifts his tie with his hand so that Esther can see it.

'Your clothes are really nice today.'

'It's nice, right. I've just bought it.'

'Also the shirt?'

'Yes.'

'See you.'

'See you next Monday.'

What I see in this peculiar interaction is a kind of psychotherapy, assuming the form of a bombardment of questions intended to identify and convert the sickness within Aziz in a way that is not unlike the conversion and expelling of the jinn in Islamic exorcisms. According to Esther, Aziz's psychotic episodes are characterised by, among other things, denial of his delusions.[4] Just as the jinn of Feisal and Abu Omar are forced to testify to the truth of God, Aziz is here made to testify to the healing effects of all the drugs he has to take. In being pushed to accept his illness and the true means of its cure, Aziz is meant to testify and submit his body to the truth of psychiatric healthcare. But like the jinn of Abu Omar and Feisal, Aziz, or the sickness within him, stubbornly resists being identified and converted. Layers of ironic answers and small lies in response to Esther's questions are set up as a defence against the effects of her words and drugs (see Scott 1990).

From Esther's point of view, we could read the situation as if his psychosis is applying the strategy of camouflage, disguising itself as a human subject. 'I'm a nice person,' it says, demanding of Esther a mutual recognition. This she must recognise, so as to continue a normal conversation, but at the same time she must ignore it in order not to be entrapped. This tricky situation parallels the main danger in all exorcism, namely when the shaykh enters into dialogue with the jinn. Even though a psychosis or a jinn may be weak in comparison to the vast power of God or psychotropic medicine, it still has the advantage of invisibility. Its power resides in remaining invisible, covering and camouflaging itself in a web of lies, false names, and false facades. In this situation Esther must avoid falling into the trap of recognising the psychosis as a human being. She must stay indifferent to its claim to common humanity and instead continue to recite the effects of psychotropic medicine: the pink tablets are for the side effects, the brown pills reduce the fat in your blood, the white pills help you to relax and sleep; it's good that you go to the gym, but don't eat cakes three times a week.

'Is this a nice tie?'

In the end Esther cannot resist the demand for recognition: 'Yes, your clothes are really nice today.' She is pressed for time by the many other patients she has to meet. She needs to get Aziz out of her office so that she can get on with her work. To her advantage, Aziz has been sentenced to take his medicine, so she can check his blood tests to see if he actually takes it. But this particular Monday it is clear she didn't succeed in making his consciousness submit to the healing effects of biomedicine. The large constellation of tablets and knowledge that Esther conjured in this meeting was crushed by Aziz's continued irony. The sickness within Aziz is strong, as also reported by the shaykhs who without much luck tried to exorcise his demons. Only during his hospitalisations and prolonged periods of fixation and forced medication did Esther feel the treatment had worked and his condition improved. This was the time when Aziz started to greet her by shaking her hand and even embraced her when she came to visit.

## God will make magic of no effect

Abu Omar lies on the carpet in his living room. Abu Bilal is sitting beside him with his right hand on Abu Omar's chest. Abu Bashir sits to the left, ready to grab Abu Omar if he starts to move. Abu Omar's wife, Umm Omar, sits behind, by his legs.

Three weeks have passed since the exorcism of Abu Omar in the mosque. After a couple of days at home, Abu Omar started attending prayers in the mosque again. When I spoke with him he was of few words but seemed happy. 'I'm much better now, thank God – *al-ḥamdu li-l-Lāh*,' he assured me. I was not convinced. There was something strained about the way he talked. Some days later, together with his family, Abu Omar decided he needed an additional exorcism.

This evening, in Abu Omar's house, the whole scene repeats itself. This time I cannot participate but have to hold the camera. It feels odd to not be able to help in any way. My shaky camera movements are caused by this uneasiness at being an observer to such a great struggle (see Scene 2 and Scene 12). It is much easier to be a participant.

'My hands are sweating and my throat is contracted,' Abu Omar says.

'You're afraid. Don't be afraid, put your trust in God.' Abu Bilal hands him a pillow from the sofa so that his head will not get hurt during the reading.

Abu Bilal initiates the exorcism with a supplication: 'I seek refuge with God, the All-Listening and All-Knowing, against the accursed demon.'

The supplication is repeated three times. Then Abu Bilal continues with the opening verse of the Quran (Surat al-Fatiha). This too is repeated three times, each time followed by 'Amen' and three short sharp exhalations.

> Praise belongs to God, Lord of the Worlds, the Lord of Mercy, the Giver of Mercy, Master of the Day of Judgment. It is You we worship; it is You we ask for help. Guide us to the straight path: the path of those You have blessed, those who incur no anger and who have not gone astray. (Quran 1: 1–7)

As the verse is repeated, Abu Bilal moves his hand over Abu Omar's chest and his recitation increases in tempo and intensity. Then he moves on to recite the first five verses of the second sura of the Quran, al-Baqara:

> Alif Lam Mim.[5] This is the Scripture in which there is no doubt, containing guidance for those who are mindful of God, who believe in the unseen, keep up prayer, and give out of what We have provided for them; those who believe in the revelation sent down to you, and in what was sent before you, those who have firm faith in the Hereafter. Such people are following their Lord's guidance and it is they who will prosper. (Quran 2: 1–5)

Abu Bilal now jumps to verse 255 of Surat al-Baqara. Various hadith describe this verse – the 'throne' verse, Ayat al-Kursi – as the most powerful in the Quran, and for this reason it is used extensively for healing and protection. The recitation further increases in volume and intensity. Abu Omar's eyes now open and his gaze moves abruptly, shifting its focus from Abu Bilal's face, his hand, then to Abu Bashir, then to the ceiling. His feet start to shake.

> God: there is no god but Him, the Ever Living, the Ever Watchful. Neither slumber nor sleep overtakes Him. All that is in the heavens and in the earth

belongs to Him. Who is there that can intercede with Him except by His leave? He knows what is before them and what is behind them, but they do not comprehend any of His knowledge except what He wills. His throne extends over the heavens and the earth; it does not weary Him to preserve them both. He is the Most High, the Tremendous. (Quran 2: 255)

After the throne verse, Abu Bilal jumps back to verse 102 of Surat al-Baqara – a passage that describes the struggle between Solomon and the jinn:

[They, the disbelievers] followed what the evil ones had fabricated about the Kingdom of Solomon instead. Not that Solomon himself was a disbeliever; it was the evil ones who were disbelievers. (Quran 2: 102)

As the first line of this verse is recited, Abu Omar's body jackknifes upward. Abu Bilal demands him to get down – *inzil taḥt* – and then repeats the recitation of verse 102 from the beginning. Abu Omar roars. Abu Bilal continues verse 102:

They taught people witchcraft and what was revealed in Babylon to the two angels Harut and Marut. Yet these two never taught anyone without first warning him, 'We are sent only to tempt – do not disbelieve.' From these two, they learned what can cause discord between man and wife, although they harm no one with it except by God's leave. They learned what harmed them, not what benefited them, knowing full well that whoever gained [this knowledge] would lose any share in the Hereafter. Evil indeed is the [price] for which they sold their souls, if only they knew. (Quran 2: 102)

Abu Omar again lies flat and silent on the floor. Abu Bilal jumps to verse 81 of Surat Yunus, which tells the story of the pharaoh who asks his magicians to present their magic to Moses: 'When they did so, Moses said, "Everything you have brought is magic and God will show it to be of no effect"' (Quran 10: 81).

The verse seems to have a strong impact on Abu Omar's jinn, who continues to push upward and roar. Abu Bilal repeats the last part again – 'God will show it to be of no effect' – while he and Abu Bashir force Abu Omar's body back down to the floor. Abu Omar's eyes are now wide open, anxious, and wild. Abu Bilal addresses the jinn directly: 'By God, testify that there's no god but God.' The jinn in Abu Omar responds only by a continued strained roaring.

'Who are you?' Abu Bilal repeats his question three times, but is only answered by growling. Then he starts to recite verse 81 again, repeating four times the passage declaring that God will make magic of no effect. At this moment Umm Omar, while holding the legs of her husband, asks me to stand up so as to frame the whole scene from above with my camera. Abu Omar's index finger on the right hand is stretched right out, just as it was during the exorcism three weeks before. His feet are vibrating wildly.

Abu Bilal finishes verse 81 and continues to verse 82 and the first half of verse 83:

> 'God does not make the work of mischief-makers right; He will uphold the Truth with His words, even if the evildoers hate it.' But no one believed in Moses except a few of his own people, for fear that Pharaoh and their leaders would persecute them. (Quran 10: 82–3)

Abu Bilal then jumps back and repeats 'God will make magic of no effect' (Quran 10: 81), at which point Abu Omar's body jerks violently again. Abu Bilal starts over at the beginning of verse 81, while Umm Omar forces the head of her husband down with her hand. Having repeated that God will make magic of no effect, Abu Bilal now jumps to Surat al-Baqara, verse 102, and the description of how it was not Solomon but the evil jinn (*shayāṭīn*) who were disbelievers. Abu Omar bends upwards, moaning and roaring at Abu Bilal. The veins at his throat and temples are pumping. His head is shaking with pent-up rage. Abu Bilal continues the recitation that describes how magic was sent by angels to humankind as a test, but how people have used magic to cause discord between spouses. While Abu Omar struggles to get free and stares wildly from Abu Bashir to Abu Bilal, the last part of the sentence about how magic cannot harm anyone except by God's leave is repeated.

## The many voices of God

The fierce struggle between Abu Bilal, Abu Bashir, Umm Omar, and that will within Abu Omar which refuses to give in to the demands of the shaykh continues for some time. Through the reading, Abu Omar's illness is inserted into the context of the grand struggle between humans and jinn that was instigated at the expulsion of humankind from the Garden of Eden, and played out afterwards in the time of Abraham, Moses, Solomon, Jesus, and Muhammad.

The insertion of divine text into Abu Omar's struggles transports the actual perceived event onto a different level. As pointed out by Webb Keane (2013: 9), writings in many religious traditions work this way, as 'semiotic transductors' through which something is transformed from one semiotic modality to another. In our case the divine text makes the invisible force of God present, which in turn aggravates and exposes the invisible jinn that occupies Abu Omar's body. Through the Quranic verses, the jinn is exposed to an all-powerful speaker who not only speaks directly in the first-person imperative to the prophets and humankind, but who is capable also of speaking through the voices of the prophets, believers, disbelievers, humans, and jinn. The jinn is pushed to recognise that it is battling not the shaykh, but the very laws of the divine, and that even this battle is not really its own, but rather a part of the larger scheme of the divine. The jinn is thereby rendered into a medium through which the battle is played out.

The voice of God interweaves through the multiple subject-positions, sometimes shifting its address and form of narrator within a single sentence. For example, this condensation or montage of speaker positions is seen when Abu Bilal proceeds to recite Surat al-Ikhlas (112), Surat al-Falaq (113), and Surat al-Nas (114). In these verses, as in many others, God addresses the Prophet directly in the first person through the Archangel Gabriel, ordering the Prophet to cite a protective supplication. God's words are then uttered through the words of the Prophet, who is also cited in the first person:

> Say, I seek refuge with the Lord of people, the Controller of people, the God of people, against the harm of the slinking whisperer – who whispers into the hearts of people – whether they be jinn or people. (Quran 114: 1–6)

The montage of speaker positions is further complicated when it is actualised in the exorcism by Abu Bilal as a protection for himself and his patient, as an accusation against the jinn, and as an order for it to give up its evil and essentially futile endeavour, succumbing instead to the will and protection of its Creator. As the ritual enunciator, Abu Bilal becomes a kind of 'third person' to the multiple and exceptional identity conjured through the recitation; a disembodied identity that is by no means confined within Abu Bilal's body, but rather flows and speaks through it as it also flows and speaks through the patient and the jinn.[6]

The recitation conjures a revelation akin to the time-image described by Deleuze. Like the time-image, the recitation of the many Quranic excerpts works to dissolve the dialectics of power played out between the shaykh, the patient, and the jinn. Thereby action and thought are delinked from the human subject, who is consequently transformed into a witness of life. Through the recitation it becomes clear that just like the words and actions of the various prophets and jinn cited in the Quran ultimately originate from God, so is it with the actual actions and utterances of the healer and his patient.

The exorcism proceeds with recitations of Surat al-Saffat, the last verses of Surat al-Baqara, Surat al-Qalam, Surat Ibrahim, Surat al-Jinn, and Surat al-Nahl. Abu Bilal addresses the jinn directly and demands that the jinn reveals its identity and origin: 'I will continue to read, until you burn. Say who you are. I swear by God that you'll say it. Testify that there's no god but God and that Muhammad is the Prophet of God. Where are you from?'

When finally Abu Bilal starts reading Surat al-Kafirun (109), followed by yet another repetition of the last three suras of the Quran (112–14), the struggle within Abu Omar comes to an end. Apparently the jinn succumbs to the pressure, and abandons the body it had possessed.

Throughout the exorcism the jinn appear to react more severely to some Quranic verses than others. *Ṣarʿ* or what Jørgen Aagaard identifies as trance seems to be both an intellectual and an emotional arousal of consciousness. Not only are the shaykh's tone and the aesthetics and intensity of the recitation important in the establishment of the state of *ṣarʿ*; the linguistic content of verses seems equally important. *Ṣarʿ* is ignited through a combined effort on the part of the shaykh to convey the emotional and verbal meanings of the Quran to the jinn and the patient.

With Abu Omar, the verse about Moses and the magicians of the Egyptian pharaoh (Quran 10: 81) appeared most successful. During the exorcism, Abu Bilal continues to return to this verse when other verses appear to be less effective. In the discussion after the exorcism it is also the visible effect of this particular verse that leads the shaykh to conclude that the root of Abu Omar's problem is not the jinn, but magic (see Scene 12). In this way the verses of the Quran work as a tool of diagnosis. In the exorcism of Feisal (discussed in Chapters 4 and 5) the verse about Solomon and the jinn (Quran 2: 102) appeared to have the greatest effect, forcing the jinn to talk and circumvent the meanings of the divine words. Like Esther's attempt to find a crack through which to find a way into the problems and suffering of Aziz, the shaykh scans the patient with the recitation of the struggles recorded in the Quran in order to locate and identify the proper cause and nature of the illness.[7]

Despite the high intensity of Abu Omar's exorcism, it is not clear to what degree the healing ritual was successful. It is a daunting task for the healer to overcome the power struggle between the patient, the jinn and himself, and often efforts do not succeed. Since the jinn is invisible, it may easily escape the healer's attacks. It only has to outsmart the healer by seducing him into conversation. As long as the healer does not read the Quran, the jinn feels safe. Furthermore the jinn may simply leave the body, and then re-enter once the healer has left the patient.

To understand the resistance of the jinn we need to imagine the enormous precarity it may feel when exposed to the Quranic verses. Just as Aziz may feel touched by the flames of hellfire when embarking on psychotropic treatment, so does the jinn, according to my interlocutors, feel the burning of the verses. During the recitation of the Quran the jinn is exposed to the vast alterity of God evoked by the polyphonic condensation of voices. Succumbing to this alterity requires it to withdraw from its illegal occupation of a human body. As Aziz must put his faith into the world of biomedicine, the jinn must take the leap out of the human body into a certitude in something that cannot be contained. During exorcisms jinn often beg shaykhs for mercy, because their kin are waiting outside the human body.

If they succumb to the will of God by taking the Islamic decree of faith (*shahāda*) and exit the body, their kin on the other side will often stand ready to kill them for their betrayal.

With Abu Omar the exorcism appeared to have some effect, but it was only partly successful. After the exorcism, Abu Bilal, Umm Omar, and Abu Bashir were speculating as to whether the jinn had died or left Abu Omar's body during his last cry. But soon after the exorcism finished, it became clear that something was still at work in his body. When Abu Bilal read Surat al-Nas above a white bowl filled with water and leaves of *sidr*, Abu Omar's right cheek started to show signs of possession and agitation (Scene 12). Several additional shaykhs performed a variety of healing rituals in subsequent months, yet Abu Omar's symptoms kept coming back. Each time, however, the exorcisms seemed to establish a moment of relief, a break from an otherwise difficult reality, and a hope that at some point all the pain would be relieved.

With Aziz, the situation is the same. He continues to be hospitalised periodically. After one severe outbreak of psychosis his medication was increased. Currently he seems relatively stable, but he complains about the side effects. His right index finger is constantly stretched upward for weeks or months at a time. He feels a restlessness and agitation inside his body. His wife complains that he sleeps all the time. When I visit him he continues to reiterate his explanation about how he has been the victim of blue magic from Turkey. I do not know what to say or propose. He knows himself, however. As he says, all the pain he suffers will be repaid if he is patient.

## Freedom in slavery

Both the exorcism of Abu Omar and the psycho-education of Aziz can be described as working through a 'cinematic' dissolution of dialectical thinking that creates the condition of mind that makes submission to an all-powerful external outside possible. From this perspective, what characterises both possession and psychosis is their illusory rootedness in a form of social narcissism that denies the real origin of illness and the only true path to healing.

In psychiatry schizophrenia and psychosis are sometimes understood to develop through forms of denial, either of the self or of the other. As described by Harrop and Trower (2003), schizophrenia usually appears during adolescence, at the moment when an emerging sense of self is most vulnerable. In neo-orthodox Islamic theology, denial of the proper relation between self and other also lies at the root of magic and possession. In a sense magic and possession, as a violation of divine law, are impossible, since they only operate by disregarding and cloaking the inevitable state of dependency on God that characterises the human condition. It is through this illusion, which can be maintained only for as long as the social does not look beyond itself, that the victim of magic and possession comes to be entrapped. The dialectical game for power only exists within the social as long as the boundaries of the social are kept intact. Once the social is opened up and reveals itself to its essentially non-social origin, the dialectic is dissolved.

In Islam, the solution to the dialectical struggle for power between humans and between humans and jinn is of course God. In psychiatry, it is the biochemical agents that may re-establish a healthy circuit of the mental processes occurring in the brain. Hence the task of the psychiatrist, the nurse, and the shaykh is to work as mediators for this realisation to occur. Through the mediation of the healer, the patient is confronted with an overpowering alterity to which resistance gives no meaning. Contrary to anthropological theories about healing that emphasise alterity primarily in the human 'other', what Danish psychiatry and Islamic exorcisms have in common is their insistence on a notion of alterity as being located entirely outside the socially human.

In suggesting this analysis I have relied on Marks and Kapferer's rethinking of religious art and ritual in terms of Deleuze's philosophy of cinema. Yet it is clear that much of Deleuze's writing points in very different directions to what I propose here. Deleuze finds in the dissolution of the subject facilitated by the time-image a suspension of the Hegelian dialectic and the propensity for rational mastery and judgement which, according to him, constantly restrict the creative potential of humans. The birth of unrestricted human creativity, seems to be the vision held by Deleuze – a point to which I will return in Chapter 7. Yet, despite Deleuze's blunt criticism of dialectical reasoning, I find his theory of cinema not so distant from the solution proposed by the early Hegel (2003[1807]) in his seminal text about lordship and bondage – a text that also became highly influential in the writings of Merleau-Ponty and Kierkegaard.

Autonomous lordship, as Hegel (2003: 112) makes clear, is impossible, since mastery only exists on the condition of its affirmation by the slave. Hence as Merleau-Ponty (1964: 68) points out, it is the slave, not the master, who holds the most exact awareness of the human situation. The slave has faced and lived through the fear of death and, in so doing, submitted his consciousness to another consciousness. Through his acceptance of death as the ultimate destination, life becomes possible. The master, on the contrary, wants to exist independently for no one but himself. Yet in order to experience independence he needs recognition of his mastery by someone who has been made subordinate to him. The master finds himself trapped in the realisation that: '[t]he truth of the independent consciousness is accordingly the consciousness of the Bondsman' (Hegel 2003: 110). Hence the slave holds the only possible mastery – the mastery that resides in realising that autonomy is impossible and that independent self-consciousness only exists insofar as it is recognised and acknowledged as such by another consciousness. Self-consciousness, for Hegel (2003: 104), thus arises when both slave and master agree to be slaves and form what he calls a 'spiritual unity in its duplication'.

What is sacrificed in this movement, described both by Hegel and, I believe, also by Deleuze in his theory of cinema, is the illusion of subjective consciousness as an independent, autonomous phenomenon. Human thought and consciousness arise, Deleuze writes, due to 'the presence of an unthinkable in thought' and 'the presence to infinity of another thinker in the thinker, who shatters every monologue of a thinking self' (2005b: 163; see also Marks 2010: 69).

In this context I understand Hegel's notion of self-consciousness as the freedom and peace of mind that can be experienced upon realising that autonomous mastery is not possible. Hegel's phenomenology parallels that of Merleau-Ponty when he describes the dependency of subjective human vision on the vast, normative, all-encompassing viewpoint that he refers to by his concept of invisibility. As Merleau-Ponty (1964: 70) points out in a critique of Sartre and Simone de Beauvoir's concept of freedom, the most complete definition of human existence is to be found 'in the idea of a universality which men [*sic*] affirm or imply by the mere fact of their being and at the very moment of their opposition to each other, in the idea of a reason immanent in unreason, of a freedom which comes into being in the act of accepting limits and to which the least perception, the slightest movement of the body, the smallest action, bear incontestable witness'. This is freedom of the kind that Kierkegaard's De Silentio speculates might have been experienced by Abraham and his son on their three-and-a-half days' ascent to the summit of Moriah – the freedom from 'freedom', or perhaps more precisely freedom from the impulse to resist, which has so often been taken as the emblematic expression of liberal autonomy in Western academia (Mahmood 2005: 10).

My claim that these thoughts by Merleau-Ponty and Deleuze, linking all the way back to Kierkegaard and Hegel, can provide a useful framework for understanding the interactions between jinn, patients, psychiatrists, and Muslim healers need further empirical evidence. Since after an exorcism, the jinn themselves are usually exterminated or disappear into the realm of the invisible, it is not really possible to retrieve from them proper statements or descriptions of their experiences during Quranic recitation (cf. Bubandt 2009). Patients who have entered the state of *ṣarʿ* normally remember very little about what has happened, and awake to consciousness in a highly confused and ambivalent condition, usually just mumbling small supplications for the help of God.

In making these claims I rely also on my own experiences while witnessing these events as a participant observer; the experience of loss of control, of witnessing phenomena beyond my perceptual and analytic capacities, of having been moved and touched by something I cannot contain. Often, however, this confusion and doubt is resolved through an almost automatic plea for guidance and protection (see also the supplications of Abu Omar in Scene 12). As Adrees phrased it in the discussion of the YouTube exorcism (see Chapter 3, Scene 7), witnessing these strange occurrences may be beneficial in that they teach people the importance of praying. Thus in the loss of control, peace of mind can be obtained. In Hegel, and as Pandolfo (2018: 206) also argues in her analysis of spiritual dispossession in Morocco, this special sense of freedom can be described as the peace enjoyed when the fatality of earthly life is accepted as one's ultimate destiny.

When I scroll through my fieldnotes and film recordings I find parallel emotional expressions for patients who did not enter the state of *ṣarʿ*. When I asked Nadia who was recited over in Scene 5 (see also Chapter 4), she described her experience like this:

'When Abu Bilal was reading, there were many emotions, but in the beginning it was a kind of fear. Just when he started to read I began to cry. I was shaking, it was just the right side. It was my right arm and right leg. And then I remember that I liked it when he was singing but despite this I was feeling really bad. I felt that he shouldn't do this. But then it became better and better. Afterwards I was crying just from joy. It was happiness in some way. So it was a mixed emotion, but in the beginning it was mainly fear and in fact it was very negative. It wasn't positive.'

In her retelling of her feelings, Nadia mentions the shaking of the right side of her body as an indication that she had been touched by a jinn – something Abu Bilal confirmed could have been the case in their conversation just after the event. Several months previous, her engagement had been broken off. She had entered a state of depression and misery, and during these months had felt unable to pray and ask for God's help. At night she had severe nightmares of being under surveillance by unknown persons. After the Quranic reading and the removal of the images in her bedroom she describes how the nightmares instantly disappeared, and how she felt 'liberated' (*befriet*) and 'almost weightless'. In addition, she described how 'I saw light, I wanted to marry again and have children'. Reading *ruqya* in the theoretical framework of Hegel, we can say that it seems to be a transformative event – a kind of 'traumatic awakening' (Pandolfo 2011; 2018) – that subordinates individual resistances in order to renew the possibility of the special kind of human mastery that resides in submitting oneself to mortality and the requirements of a mortal and morally good life – in this case the morality implied in reproduction through marriage and parenthood.

A young man diagnosed with schizophrenia had a different experience with *ruqya*. For a long time he strongly resisted medical treatment as both he and his relatives were convinced that jinn were at the root of his problem, and that for this reason medical treatment with psychotropics was not necessary but potentially dangerous. At one point a Quranic reading was organised. Several family members were gathered. He was made to stand up, while the shaykh put his right hand on his forehead and started to recite. The young man described the anxiety he felt standing there, thinking about how suddenly the jinn would come out and speak through his mouth. At some point in the reading he collapsed and fell to the floor. His relatives and the shaykh quickly gathered around him. He remembered how he had looked up into their faces, bewildered by the fact he had just realised that 'It's just me, it isn't a jinn'. The *ruqya* made him and his family realise that since it was not jinn related, he had to embark on psychiatric medication, and that this was an obligation. Once he had accepted the biomedical nature of his condition and the religious necessity of taking psychotropic medication, his condition finally began to improve.

What happens then in the consultation between Aziz and his nurse Esther? In Hegel's terms, Esther seems to be in the position of the master, who despite being backed up by all the power of psychiatric healthcare and juridical assistance, and despite the fact that the patient does take the medication (or at least part of it), still cannot get her patient fully to submit his consciousness to the treatment. Aziz's sickness is beyond her reach. This Monday, Esther, Aziz, and his psychosis remain trapped within the Hegelian dialectic. Despite the overwhelming assemblage of pills and psychiatric knowledge she presents, it is not enough. Her authority is crumbling, precisely because it is unable to attach to that greater authority of biomedicine. Her evocation of this external knowledge does not succeed in overpowering the patient. Instead it points towards the healer and shows a weakness.

If Aziz's powers of resistance remain intact in Scene 8, then something else seems to happen in the last scene of the film, which was recorded in autumn 2011 (Scene 14). On that day, representatives from the social services (*Livsværkstederne*) and the police were gathered together with Jørgen and Esther to assess Aziz's condition and ongoing treatment. In several ways the situation resembles the exorcism of Abu Omar. Aziz is surrounded by a group of people, all of whom direct their gaze at him, ask him questions, and present their understanding of his present condition and the reasons he needs continued medication.

The practice of gathering representatives from all the welfare institutions involved in the treatment of mentally ill patients has become increasingly popular in recent years. 'Integrated treatment', as it is often called, builds on the idea that it is necessary to consider the 'whole' human being in order to facilitate a process of recovery (see also Chapter 4). The idea of a human as ideally being whole might be regarded as the quintessential requirement of Western individualism – i.e. the human understood as indivisible and autonomous. Wholeness, however, is by no means what characterises the experience of all human beings. Indeed we can observe the fracture which occurs at the moment we utter the idea that 'I am me'. As Hegel and others have made clear, the human experience is often characterised by a high degree of separateness, the experience of 'I' not always being 'me' (see Nielsen, Mikkelsen, and Aagaard 2009). This might also be the case at the onset of serious disturbances such as psychosis, depression, schizophrenia, or jinn possession. Suffering is arguably part of the experience of not being whole.

It may be that integrated treatment works simply because the communication between health professionals from different disciplines allows for a better understanding and a more holistic approach to the treatment of patients. Yet we also need to consider how the mere presence of several healers facing a patient has in itself an overpowering effect. The holism of monotheistic religions such as Christianity or Islam, but perhaps also of modern biomedical science, can be seen as offering a whole to which a patient might seek to reattach. Perhaps some of the success of 'integrated treatment' can also be understood in its ability to conjure such a whole – a holy or sacred space with which the patient may aspire to be reunited.

As in the case of Abu Omar, Aziz is observed through a number of different lenses – criminal, social, psychiatric, and on this particular occasion even anthropological and cinematic. In this situation we all sit around him, representing this whole, staring at him from all sides. Esther could not do this alone, not even when she invoked the power of all the medications of Aziz's treatment. Today, however, she is not alone, but accompanied by four other people.

'Do you think you have problems?' Jørgen asks Aziz. Aziz immediately denies that he has any problems, but Jørgen is persistent, 'Not at all, no problems? … Do you remember why you were sentenced to treatment?'

'A couple of times you have been a bit agitated,' says Esther. 'Should I see this as a good or a bad sign?'

'Today you appear to be feeling very well,' says Birte, Aziz's social worker. 'But sometimes I've been worried. Sometimes you've been troubled. Sometimes you haven't been well.'

Finally Aziz succumbs to the pressure. He gives in and confesses: 'We can't be well all the time. I have many problems inside. All people have problems. No one can be happy all the time.' At this moment he is unable to resist the pressure any longer. An atmosphere of relief fills the room. Apparently, at this moment, Aziz has finally become a patient.

## *Notes*

1 Neither Hegel nor Marx directly phrased their concepts of the 'dialectic' in terms of thesis, antithesis, and synthesis in their work. Rather, these distinctions were elaborated by Johann Fichte (see Kaufmann 1965).

2 For more details see e.g. Eli Lilly: http://pi.lilly.com/us/zyprexa-pi.pdf; US Food and Drug Administration: www.drugs.com/zyprexa.html (retrieved 22 April 2019).

3 The public and scholarly debate about Olanzapine is extensive (see also Levine 2004; Ray et al. 2009: 230). On several occasions Eli Lilly has been accused for not disclosing their findings of adverse effects, illegal marketing, and ghost writing. Between 2006 and 2007, Eli Lilly agreed to pay at least 1.2 billion USD to settle approximately 28,500 lawsuits from people claiming to be suffering from side effects such as diabetes or other diseases that the company had initially tried to deny (see Berenson 2007). In 2009 Eli Lilly admitted guilt and agreed to pay 1.415 billion USD to settle the criminal charge of marketing Zyprexa for un-approved uses, including dementia, depression, anxiety, irritability, aggression, hostility, sleep, and mood disorders (US Department of Justice 2009). In Denmark, Eli Lilly was sued by Mikkel Dorph, who developed diabetes and later died of an untreated insulin shock. Contrary to the US authorities, the Danish Patient Insurance Association claimed diabetes to be an 'acceptable side-effect' for people treated with Zyprexa (Rasmussen 2006: 18–19).

4 See Luhrmann (2000: 140) for a description of how patients' denials of illness or desires to end treatment are frequently understood as symptoms of illness.

5 These are three Arabic letters. Various theories speculate on their meaning, but Muslim scholars mainly agree that they signify the existence of a knowledge beyond human comprehension.

6 Carlo Severi (2002: 35) describes a strikingly similar speaker identity at work in American Indian Shamanism, whereby healers become 'third-persons' to a disembodied enunciator speaking through them in a way that entirely short-cuts time and physical space. During fieldwork I followed a number of Somali healers who practise a joint form of *ruqya* that even more directly conveyed the conglamerate of perspectives and voices in the Quran. By sitting in a circle around the patient, they would each recite different parts of the Quran until the entire text had been read, conjuring thereby an almost indecipherable cacophony of voices.

7 A traditional Morroccan healer quoted by Pandolfo (1997: 142) describes the process of healing through Quranic recitations as a form of X-raying. Yet like Abu Bilal, this healer emphasises that 'unlike what happens with X rays, we cannot see the jinns directly. [I] can only guess their shape in smoke, or in the shadows [*khayāl*] … There must always be a *wasiṭa*, an intermediary, a link, a term between: for if the jinns appeared right in front of me they'd put me in a state of fitna: I would be seized by madness'. See also Steven Friedson (1996) for a parallel analysis of drumming among the Tumbuka of Malawi as a tool of diagnosis that ignites the spirits and forces them to explain why they have possessed a person.

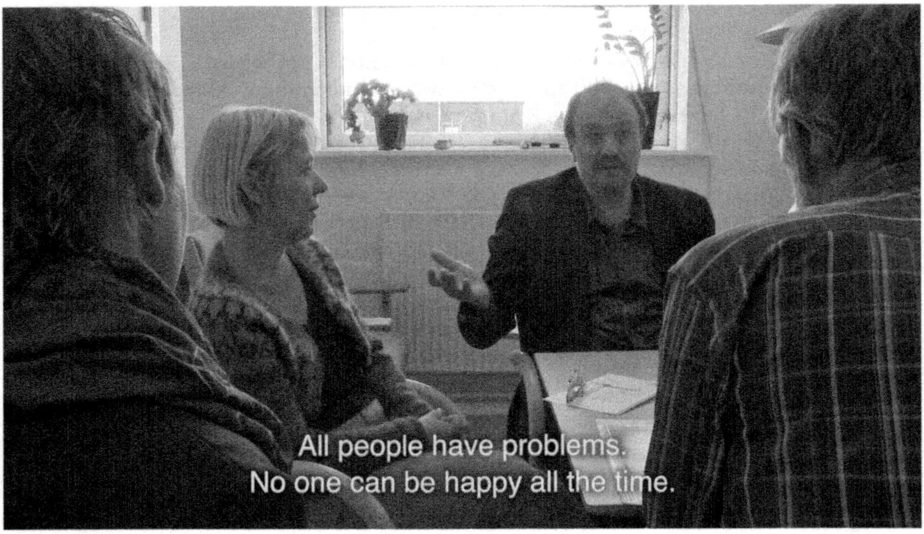
All people have problems.
No one can be happy all the time.

7.1 Still from Scene 14

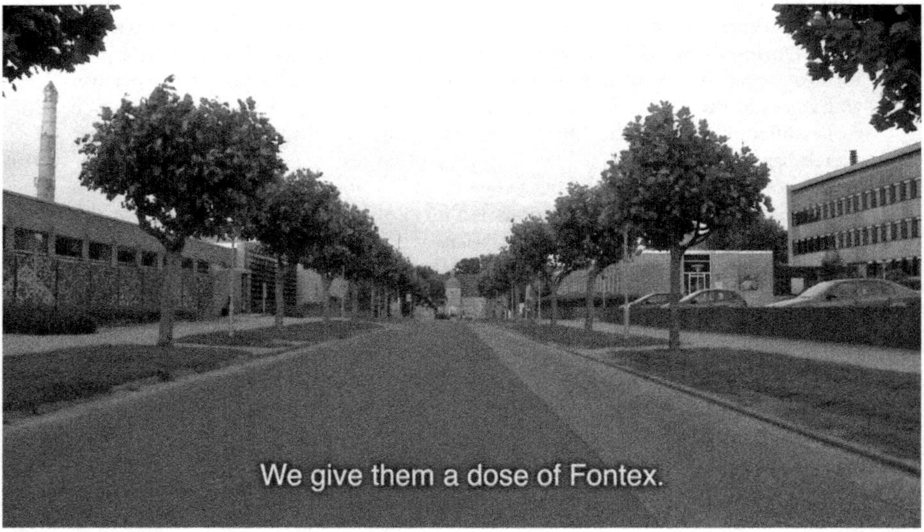
We give them a dose of Fontex.

7.2 Still from Scene 13

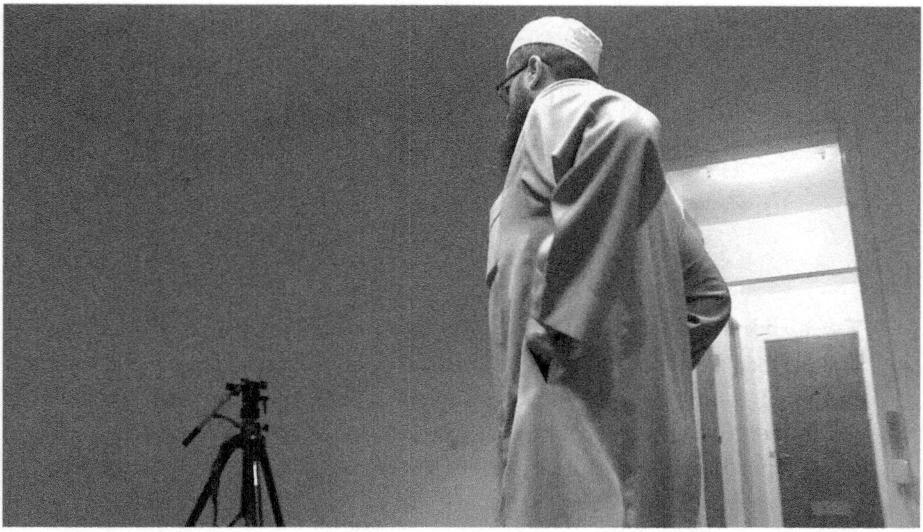

7.3 Still from Scene 12

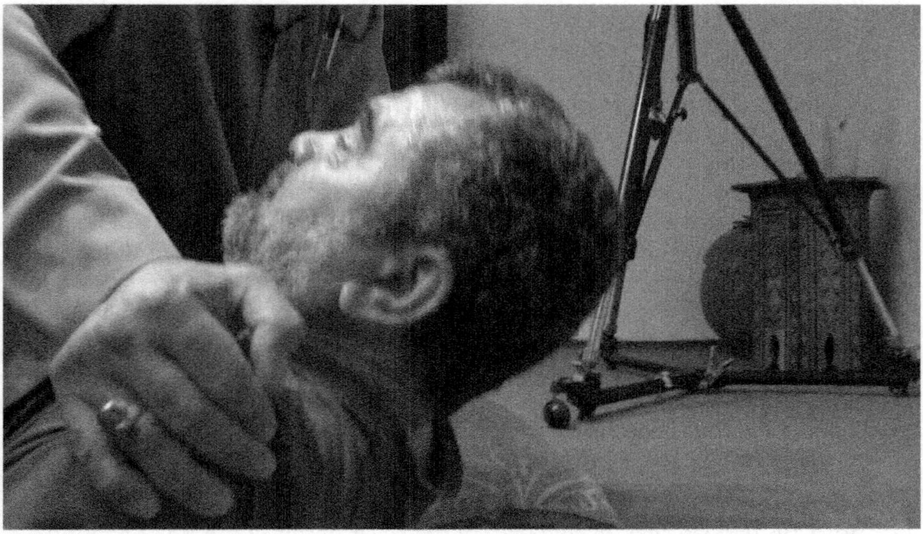

7.4 Still from Scene 2

# 7

# No healing here

In a short fictional story, the Argentinian writer Jorge Luis Borges has described how one of his acquaintances, Carlos Argentino, once invited him to his house to see a small iridescent globe called the Aleph, which was hidden under a step of the stairway to the cellar. In looking at it, all possible perspectives in the universe were revealed in one gigantic instant:

> The Aleph's diameter was probably little more than an inch, but all space was there, actual and undiminished. Each thing (a mirror's face, let us say) was infinite things, since I distinctly saw it from every angle of the universe. I saw the teeming sea; I saw the daybreak and nightfall; I saw the multitudes of America; I saw a silvery cobweb in the centre of a black pyramid; I saw a splintered labyrinth (it was London); I saw, close up, unending eyes watching themselves in me as in a mirror; I saw all the mirrors on earth and none of them reflected me; I saw in a backyard of Soler Street the same tiles that thirty years before I'd seen in the entrance of a house in Fray Bentos; I saw bunches of grapes, snow, tobacco, lodes of metal, steam; I saw convex equatorial deserts and each one of their grains of sand; I saw a woman in Inverness whom I shall never forget; I saw her tangled hair, her tall figure, I saw the cancer in her breast; [...] I saw the drawer of a writing table (and the handwriting made me tremble), unbelievable, obscene, detailed letters, which Beatriz had written to Carlos Argentino; I saw a monument I worshipped in the Chacarita cemetery, I saw the rotted dust and bones that had once deliciously been Beatriz Viterbo; I saw the circulation of my dark blood; I saw the coupling of love and the modification of death; I saw the Aleph from every point and angle, and in the Aleph I saw the earth; I saw my own face and my own bowels; I saw your face; and I felt dizzy and wept, for my eyes had seen that secret and conjectured object whose name is common to all men but which no man has looked upon – the unimaginable universe. (Borges 1971: 27–9)

What Borges describes having seen in the cellar of this house is not a vision common to everyone. Rather, it is the vision of God's eye, the view from everywhere. Relieved from human perspectival seeing, this vision presents itself as supreme and absolute objectivity. This strange and impossible viewpoint is what Merleau-Ponty in his discussion of object perception has defined as the normative viewpoint from which all other viewpoints deviate. Borges's story continues, however, with the problems of how to account for such omnipresent perception within the confines of human language. Regardless of how hard he tries, it is impossible to contain this vision and write it down. In the pursuit of capturing it, both Borges and his friend are driven to the verge of madness.

A year after Borges has seen the Aleph, he notes how he began to speculate whether the Aleph's revelation of the entirety of the universe could have been a fraud. He tries to recall how he – while looking at the Aleph – perhaps in glimpses saw several other Alephs hidden in different places around the world. This leads him to wonder whether these Alephs could have revealed visions even more complete than the vision he did in fact see, but which he at the time of writing had almost forgotten. With time, the memories he has of this sublime revelation begin to dissolve in favour of grey spots of doubt and uncertainty. Regardless of whether he did actually see the universe in its entirety, his limited memory does not allow him to keep this total vision through time. Rather than total objectivity, his memory of the Aleph becomes a partial narrative comprised of what he remembers best. In a vicious act of jealousy, Borges decides to deny having seen the Aleph in Carlos Argentino's cellar, hoping to transmit his own uncertainty to his acquaintance as well.

Borges's story may in this context serve as a warning pointing to the impossibility of total vision and total objectivity. The jealous attempt by Borges to transfer his own doubt about the truth-value of the Aleph to Carlos Argentino by denying having seen it may serve as another warning. Regardless of whether Borges did truly witness the complete revelation of the universe, the knowledge he obtained is immediately used against his acquaintance in their mutual rivalry. This story about the revelation of the truth of the universe therefore also tells a story about the way human knowledge is always limited and shaped by our various desires and agendas.

This issue has also been extensively debated within the discipline of anthropology. The realisation that all knowledge and scientific enquiry are necessarily biased and often carry more-or-less conscious agendas led many anthropologists to a crisis of representation and to a rejection of the traditional anthropological knowledge project (see e.g. Clifford and Marcus 1986). Rather than a 'neutral' investigation of the human condition, claims were made that the discipline needed to be reframed as an emancipatory project. However, as Haraway (1991) has forcefully argued, it is only by accepting the fact that all human knowledge is situated that we may continue our investigations, which will never lead us to the objective layout of the sociocultural worlds we live in, but which may lead to situated and – in this sense – partially objective accounts of them.

In this present context, we may seem to have built up a conglomerate of analytical arguments and perspectives not entirely dissimilar to the vision described by Borges. While weaving in and out of Islamic exorcisms and psychiatry I have considered these treatments from multiple sides and angles.

It seems as if these perspectives and the multiple and often disconnected fragments that constitute the experience of fieldwork have come to fit as nuts and bolts within an overall theoretical framework – an argument about exorcism and psychiatry as being essentially about the same thing, namely the dissolution, sacrifice, and submission of the human subject to an all-encompassing external structuring. If such a finite scheme of analytical thought has been attributed to the worlds of others, then somewhere along the way I must have left behind the ethical writing propagated by writers such as Levinas and Merleau-Ponty (see Chapters 1 and 3).

Skimming through my notebooks and the many hours of film material, I am sometimes drawn towards other visions and opportunities that never reached the editing table or the pages of this book. Small details in images remind me of the worlds of vision and knowledge I simply overlooked in my eagerness to convey those particular stories and images discussed in the preceding chapters.

To be sure, any work of film and writing will always involve such sacrifices of visibility. As both Taussig (1999) and Latour (2002) have taught us, and as described in Chapter 4, to build or present an image often requires the destruction or defacement of other images. But this research project was not about creating a new all-encompassing visibility. It was about invisibility, *al-ghayb*, that which cannot be seen, and the way in which that which cannot be seen always lurks in the shadows or in the edges of our gaze, dragging us towards ever further degrees of invisibility. I wish to dedicate this concluding chapter to four such dissonant 'Aleph'-like figures that still stick out as pockets of invisibility pointing towards other possible interpretations than the ones I have been able to contain within the analysis so far.

First I will take an alternative look at the oscillation between doubt and faith among the nurses in psychiatric healthcare. Then I will consider a tripod that Umm Omar kindly provided for me to film the exorcism of her husband, but which I refused to use. Thirdly I wish to expand the conclusions we may draw from the joining of ritual, cinematic montage, and Deleuze's notion of the time-image, especially with regard to what happens beyond the time-image. Finally, I will close with a description of a short video sequence, presented to me by Abu Bilal, of Feisal lying on the carpet of his flat in a pool of blood and vomit – a video which I was shown so I could see the real power of *ruqya* and the dark substance of magic when it has left its victim.

## Doubt and faith

To take seriously other people's reality is, as outlined in Chapter 2, by no means an easy task. In addition to a conceptual rearrangement of thoughts and presuppositions, it may sometimes also require a rather fundamental disruption of one's own perceptual and emotional faculties. Such disruption is not necessarily difficult to achieve, but it may be difficult to deal with. Prolonged fieldwork, in the sense of actual participation in whatever practices people are engaging in, seems to be the key methodological tool in order to achieve this disruption. The longer and more intensely one participates in other people's lives, the better the chances one will be touched by them. More than 'observation' or 'qualitative interviewing', active 'participation' in the fullest sense of the word is arguably the most fundamental generator and transformer of anthropological knowledge (Stoller 1984; Turner 1993, 2006; Otto 1997).

Throughout my fieldwork I would shift contexts abruptly, often several times a day, between Islamic healing rituals and lectures on God's demands on our daily conduct in the mosques, discussions about the social construction of truth among colleagues in the Department of Anthropology at Aarhus University, and heart-breaking attempts by nurses in the psychiatric institutions to convince their patients to take their antipsychotic drugs. As the months and years proceeded it became increasingly difficult not to bring back experiences from the field to my private life, my dreams, and my common-sensical ways of perceiving the world.

The fractured experiences of shifting contexts, languages, vocabulary, bodily behaviour, and emotional as well as perceptual dispositions may have been part of the reason I became particularly attuned to similarities between the Islamic and psychiatric approaches to healing, even when, on the contrary, many of the practitioners tried to make me recognise their differences. My desire to show these similarities derived both from a wish to unsettle some prejudices between believers of the two different systems of treatment, but also from a necessity within my own mind to assemble a whole out of the particular kind of ruptures I experienced in the field. All analysis of human life is situated, as Haraway (1991) points out, not just politically and theoretically, but also in the much more basic sense of being a part of someone's life. Any analysis arises out of the life of the researcher, and in one way or another, reflects it. I do not think this bias invalidates analysis. It is by no means to deny a commitment to objectivity, but it is an acknowledgement of the fact that objectivity can only be approached by recognising our limited access to it.

In this book I have proposed the argument that somehow doubt was the indispensable requirement for the sacrificial acts of faith required by healers and patients during procedures of both psychiatric and Islamic healing (see Chapters 4 and 5). Here I wish to discuss an asymmetry that I have not yet properly addressed. Doubt does not function in exactly the same ways and to the same degrees in the two systems of treatment. Whereas the Muslim healers appear to sincerely believe in God, the same cannot always be said of psychiatrists and nurses with regard to the main component of their healing, namely psychotropic medicine. While doubt prevails at all levels of treatment in the Islamic case – except regarding the ontological reality of God – doubt sweeps through the corridors of the psychiatric institutions, and even penetrates far into the production of so-called evidence-based medicine. Indeed, if we were to fully assimilate the power of biomedicine with the Islamic concept of God, we would have to regard many of these psychiatric health professionals as heretics.

When I first presented my project to the nurses in the psychiatric institutions, their first response was to tell me I had gone to the wrong place: 'There is no healing here' (see Chapter 2). In this book I have taken this odd response as an expression of the form of doubt – 'the movement of resignation' as Kierkegaard would call it – preceding and constituting the necessary condition for a leap into faith. Understood in this way, 'no healing here' could be seen not as pejorative of Danish psychiatric healthcare as such, but rather as a positive expression of a view of healing as an ideal gift that is always and necessarily received from elsewhere (Ohnuma 2007: 149). In other words, 'no healing here' was part of the defacement required for accessing the space of the sacred as an always deferred truth beyond the reach of human perception or agentive capacity (Taussig 1999). As we have seen, in some ways these statements by the nurses parallel those of the shaykhs disclaiming their powers to heal (see Chapter 4).

Yet there could be other ways of understanding the apparently pessimistic statements by nurses. What if the doubt they expressed was not seen as the necessary fuel required to perform the leap of faith? What if, rather, their doubt was expressive of an entirely different belief or certitude, not in the power of biomedicine, but in the human capacity for care and self-healing?

Several nurses expressed their regrets about how what they saw as the core of their healing profession, namely human care, was being thinned out by the increasing amount of time they had to spend as secretaries for the distribution, documentation, and keeping of protocols of their patients' consumption of psychotropic medicine. Recall the nurse cited in Chapter 2:

'I can't just tell the patient that I don't understand the medicine and that I wouldn't dare to take it myself. Shouldn't we go to the cinema once a week instead? … We have our key tasks: to diagnose and to find the correct medication. Medication, this is the guys who get the money, this is where you have evidence. Nobody receives money for the soft things, here there's no evidence, it's just stuffing. But for me to establish a relationship of trust is the most important.'

Esther also seems to express something along these lines when she re-evaluates her views on Islamic healing in Scene 13:

'I don't think that our medications are always the most appropriate. Many of the basic existential problems that cause people to suffer – we try to medicate them. Perhaps we need the intimacy of a sweat lodge more. Understand me correctly. Some people are so ill that they become dangerous. But all those who sat on a cold potty in their childhood or ended up in family or work relations that make life difficult and make them sad – then I just don't know. Don't you think the intimacy and care that the Navajos could give in a sweat lodge would be just as healing? Then the whole society knows that something is not working here. I'm not well, take care of me for a while. We give them a dose of Fontex.'

Throughout the book I have discussed the similarities between Islamic exorcism and psychiatric healthcare – two systems of treatment which both rely heavily on the invocation of invisible healing agents external to the domain of the social. Yet in our conversation, Esther might also be pointing towards a different analytical scheme – one in which the similarities lie not between psychotropic medication and Islamic exorcisms, but between the forms of human care provided by a range of 'traditional' and 'religious' healing practices around the world – care that is intimately tied to the social and arises primarily through the re-establishment of social relationships and trust in the world. In Esther's re-evaluation of the Islamic treatment, she highlights the way in which Abu Bilal touches his patient, and the musicality and even kindness of his voice when reciting the Quran. What Esther notices is not the transgressive, even sacrificial, interventions I have been describing, but the element of care, perhaps even the caress expressed by the exorcism. For Esther, this contrasts with much of her own treatment. Indeed this is what she wishes she had the time to give to her patients, but more often than not she finds she has simply become a secretary to the biomedical industry and the bureaucracy of Danish healthcare. As she also said: 'We can easily remove or dampen a psychosis with the medication. But sometimes I feel we leave a void in the patient.' By contrast she sees in the exorcism a situation in which the healer removes a destructive force from the body of the patient, but afterwards the patient is 're-filled' by touch, words, and blessed water. 'When does it become dangerous?' asks Esther, 'Perhaps this is when you leave a void. But this isn't what this shaykh does. He fills something into the void.'

Esther might here be pointing to a type of analysis that would align the humanist project of healing as compassionate care with the Islamic exorcisms as well as the use of sweat lodges among the Navajo people in the American Midwest. In this she would be close to the model of healing proposed both by Turner (1992; 2006) and also by anthropologists such as Whyte (1997), Mattingly (1998), and Callan (2012). She would be pointing towards a form of humanism, not necessarily based in the liberal, secular idea of the individual as a self-possessed autonomous entity, but rather of the 'pre-modern' kind described by Mattingly (2012). Against Foucault's interpretation of the Aristotelian 'virtue ethics' that emphasises the 'human' as the effect of particular technologies of the self, Mattingly (2012: 164) argues for a pragmatic, decidedly 'humanist' virtue ethics that recognises the vulnerability and uncertainty of life, but which also sees human existence as an open-ended process through which individual action and judgement is not only a possibility but a constant necessity required by the ambiguity of life.

Like Mattingly, Esther seems not to be positing the much-detested liberal, secular notion of 'self-sufficient humanism'. Rather she might quite simply be pointing to a notion of 'self-healing' as a fundamentally social process, through which individuals may act together to provide a shelter for one another against misfortune (see also Whyte 1997). In so doing, Esther would also be aligning herself with the many medical anthropologists, physicians, and social theoreticians currently engaged in criticising the regime of psychopharmacology. This critique is encapsulated by Healy (2006) in his study of how a system of biomedical trials, originally intended merely as an introductory test against placebo, became generalised as the stamp par excellence of psychopharmacological efficiency. As he writes:

> … the current evidence-based bandwagon is as hegemonic as the Freudian paradigm ever was. The result from trials are incorporated into algorithms and protocols which increasingly define a supposedly rational medicine … Evidence-based medicine sees itself as building a value-free, timeless, ahistorical science. One of the current challenges facing the history and sociology of modern medicine is to outline the origins of this belief system and the factors that maintain it. (Healy 2006: 78–9)

The arguments against the hegemony of the biomedical industry put forward by nurses, anthropologists, theoreticians, and physicians are to a large extent shared by many of my Muslim interlocutors. Like Healy, these Muslims would phrase their critique within the idiom of religious belief, yet their way of doing so is often rather more explicit. Indeed, people such as Abu Samir and Abu Bilal would even identify blind faith in the efficacy of biomedicine as a form of heretic veneration, idolatrous worship of a false god (Scene 9; see also Steinbock 2007: 16). Here I cannot help but draw a parallel between the statements of my Muslim interlocutors and Taussig's (1980) seminal study of Colombian miners and plantation workers who, living on the fringes of the global economic system, were able to look into it and see certain mischievous mechanisms at work. What they saw was oppression and exploitation, a form of commodity fetishism basically driven by greed. For Taussig's miners and plantation workers, this was their definition of the devil – the destructive and anti-social power of evil that sought to alienate humans from their immediate relations and from the commodities they produced. When my Muslim interlocutors evoke the figure of *shayṭān* as a 'power of the false' at work in the psychiatric system, and when the nurses evoke the figure of 'Medication, this is the guys who get the money', then I think they are pointing towards a diagnosis similar to the one put forward by the Colombian miners and plantation workers in Taussig's study.

I cannot count the amount of times people have asked me about the amount of money Muslim shaykhs might receive for carrying out an exorcism. These questions express the healthy suspicion of possible forgery that one should probably always consider before submitting one's body to any regime of treatment. While it is true that some shaykhs demand an amount of money to perform *ruqya*, it is also clear that within little more than half a century, psychopharmacology has grown to become a multibillion-dollar industry. The scale of revenue generated from psychotropic medication cannot be by any means compared to the gifts and payment received by some Muslim shaykhs. Despite all claims for the evidence-based foundation of psychopharmacological treatment, enough scholars have documented the problems of industry bias, fraud, ghost writing, manipulation, and silencing of negative trials for us to at least pause and concern ourselves with the question of this industry's claim to objective scientific truth. The scandals that continue to haunt Eli Lilly's olanzapine-based antipsychotics – given to Aziz in Scene 8 – provide perhaps the most extreme disclosure of industrial manipulation and fraud (see Chapter 6; Levine 2004; Healy 2006; Rasmussen 2006; Berenson 2007; Ray et. al. 2009; US Department of Justice 2009).

In this small-scale qualitative study I have had no intention of judging the efficacy of either psychiatric treatment or Islamic exorcism. Yet I have become increasingly troubled by the frustration that not only patients, but equally psychiatric nurses expressed over the various problems with psychopharmacological treatment – a frustration which for some led to such stress and dissatisfaction that they themselves became ill. For some nurses, frustration seemed to stem from thinking of the medicine they prescribe not at all as the product of 'a value-free, timeless, ahistorical science' (Healy 2006: 79), but rather as a result of the malign work of concealed capital interests. Since their criticisms seemed to never really be effectuated in action or in outright rejection of psychotropic treatment, but instead were often countered or directly contradicted by positive statements uttered by the same nurses in other contexts, I chose to understand these statements through Kierkegaard's framework, as a necessary yet paradoxical requirement of faith. In so doing I placed my main emphasis on the practices of the nurses and the certitude they appear to invest in psychiatric medication in their consultations with patients (see Chapters 2, 4, and 6). However, to take the contradictory statements of these nurses seriously might also suggest a much more critical view of modern psychiatry.

In the Islamic case the existence of doubt is a fact and even a sign of life, it is a sign that the struggle encapsulated by the notion of *jihād al-nafs*, the struggle of the self, is taking place (see also Pandolfo 2018). Doubt is what in a sense enables the possibility of faith as an active submission of one's trust to the divine (*al-tawakkul 'alā Allāh*). As Abu Bilal puts it, there would be no meaning to the divine test if there was only certitude (*'ayn al-yaqīn*, see also Chapter 1; Schielke 2010). Yet there is a tipping point. One needs to struggle against doubt. If doubt becomes too pervasive, it will result in a situation of hopelessness and abandonment of faith.

When some of the nurses I worked with realised that the bureaucratic load occupying their working days was making them ill, and when they realised they were not themselves willing to take psychopharmacological drugs, then we come close to such a tipping point; a situation in which scepticism and critique no longer serves to reproduce the system in which the nurses are embedded, and where faith in psychopharmacological treatment is gradually replaced by rejection and resistance. I believe Foucault (1982: 781), in his call for struggles that 'assert the right to be different' against the 'government of individualization', would have appreciated their defiance. The capacity of humans for resistance against oppression might also have been expressed in the following case.

## Umm Omar's tripod

Just before the second exorcism in Abu Omar's apartment – the exorcism featured in Scene 2 and described in Chapter 6 – his wife, Umm Omar, who is a trained wedding photographer, set up her large Manfrotto tripod for me. She placed it just beside her husband's head, to the right of their large television set. I thanked her for providing this piece of equipment, but it annoyed me immensely. I wanted to get a 'clean' shot of the exorcism, undisturbed by objects such as tripods, camera bags, or lighting gear. Despite my reservations about the kind of salvage anthropology inherent in some schools of ethnographic filmmaking, the auto-realist hidden inside me could not help but separate objects that did not seem 'real' or 'authentic' to the setting. Here we were, about to film an Islamic exorcism. Somewhere deep within my consciousness I 'knew' that an exorcism should have nothing to do with modern cameras or tripods. Perhaps it had everything to do with it. At least it seemed almost impossible to frame the image in such a way that the tripod would not intrude into the frame.

What was it that Umm Omar wanted me to film from up there on that tripod? As Gregory Bateson put it, in a dialogue with Margaret Mead, 'a dead camera on top of a bloody tripod … sees nothing' (Mead and Bateson 1977: 79). Mead insisted on the opposite argument. The recordings of a camera in the hands of a cameraman were useless, since the human selection of shots and angles obstructed the camera's objective access to pro-filmic reality. According to Mead, cameras should be placed on tripods or else their footage could at best be described as 'art' – useless for analytic purposes.

Art, Bateson replied, is not a term of abuse, emphasising how a selection is always made, regardless of whether the camera is placed on a tripod or is in the hands of a filmmaker. According to him, nothing objective of pro-filmic reality could be extracted in any direct, unpolluted way with a camera or any other mechanical recording device. For Bateson, the difference between a handheld camera and tripod shooting was merely the degree of freedom and creative expression.

When I set out to shoot the exorcism of Abu Omar I entirely agreed with Bateson. Cameras should not be on tripods. Except for a few interviews and b-roll shots of environments, most of the rushes I had shot for the film were handheld. I wanted to be able to move, to be free to make close-ups and full shots, to get into the action, to get the feel of the situation. I wanted footage through which I could re-express reality, and for this I needed shots that expressed people's interaction. I didn't think much about this before shooting the scene of Abu Omar, but it was definitely there in the back of my mind. I needed close-ups, medium shots, establishing shots, and reaction shots. I needed beads of sweat, a fragment of a wrenched mouth, close-ups of the feet. I needed all of this to seduce the viewer into the sense of 'being there', feel the weight and intensity of the situation, gradually building it up through longer shots, then shorter shots, then a climax of some sort. Surely I was on autopilot, part of me bent on documenting 'real' exorcism without interfering elements such as tripods, while another part of me was controlled by the unremitting repetition of Hollywood-style continuity editing with which I, like perhaps most of us, have been force-fed since I was able to focus on a television screen. In no way could I use the cold, disengaged long shots made by a camera fastened to a heavy tripod 1 metre away and 1.7 metres above the situation.

But what could the camera have seen from up here? What was it that Umm Omar wanted me to film? Was she, like Mead, concerned with the purity and indexical objectivity of the record? The handheld shooting style I embarked on was not her preferred choice. She wanted this scene recorded and seen, but not in the way I wanted to do it. She was not concerned about the intensity of the shooting, close-ups, or the creative possibilities in the subsequent editing. She was concerned that the camera should be placed where it would be able to observe and record the situation in its entirety.

As a consequence of my autopilot style of shooting, and my lack of willingness and flexibility, I will never be able to discover what the camera might have made me see from up on that tripod. I even succeeded in almost eliminating the presence of the tripod from the frame of the camera. But in each and every shot where the tripod does appear, despite my efforts to keep it out of the frame, I am reminded of the steady, bird's-eye view – Umm Omar's preferred view – that I did not allow to intrude into my film.

In addition to the tripod, other strange things happened that night. After the exorcism, I had a conversation with Umm Omar. She tried to demonstrate for me how, if I insisted on using a handheld camera, that I should at least learn certain techniques for steady handholding. I was exhausted by filming and did not pay enough attention. Then she talked about the story of her husband, how the jinn had been an ongoing problem for years, and how the jinn would sometimes release its rage on her. She spoke both in Danish and in the Iraqi dialect of Arabic, so I wasn't able to understand many of the details, but I was filming the conversation and looking forward to having a proper translation of the whole thing. When I got home the recording of our conversation had disappeared. Out of more than 100 hours of footage, this was the only recording that was ever corrupted. I tried in a number of different ways to retrieve the lost data from the memory card, but it was gone. Nothing to restore – just blank space filling the card with corrupted inaccessible data. As it turned out, I never succeeded in having a deep discussion like this with her again. In general my fieldwork became biased towards the world of men due to the segregation of sexes in these communities; it was largely inappropriate for me to spend much time talking with the wives of the men I worked with.

Nevertheless, I did hear through Abu Bilal a couple of things about the rage of the jinn that Umm Omar had described to me. A week before it all broke out in the mosque, an incident occurred during a prayer. Erdam's brother, who normally doesn't attend the prayers, had been persuaded to come to the mosque. He had been standing next to Abu Omar during the prayer, but with a small distance between his foot and Abu Omar's. The particular approach to prayer followed in the mosque prescribes that there should be no distance between people in the prayer rows. The feet should touch so as to prevent *shayāṭīn* from entering between the believers, confusing them, and dragging their attention away from God with their vicious whisperings. When this new attendee lined up in the prayer row next to Abu Omar but without placing his foot immediately adjacent to Abu Omar's foot, Abu Omar had resolutely gripped his leg and dragged it close to his foot. The man moved his leg back to the distance he thought was proper, but Abu Omar was determined, and dragged their legs close together again. After the prayer, Abu Omar strongly criticised the man for his lack of knowledge and respect: 'What kind of prayer is this?'

Abu Bilal explained to me that this is by no means proper behaviour towards a newcomer and that this was not how Abu Omar would normally behave. Obviously one should attempt to teach and help a brother perform the best possible prayer, but not in this way. 'Something aggressive is inside him. I had seen it a long time ago,' Abu Bilal said.

When I look at some of the other stories of jinn possession, a similar pattern can be discerned. In the period before the outbreak of Aziz's possession, both Aziz and his nurse Esther had explained how he had become fiercely religious. He would even go so far as to condemn the shaykhs for not being real believers. Aziz explained that he could somehow feel the jinn building up inside. When he felt this he would often try to fight it by doing a very large number of voluntary prayers and by intensively reading the Quran. Yet sometimes these attempts to build a defence against the jinn got out of hand and he found himself in situations where he could not distinguish between the will of the jinn and his own attempts to fight it.

Khalid, who was possessed by Abu Hassan (see Chapter 5), had a comparable but more complicated story. For some time Khalid had regarded his occupant jinn as a protective guardian, even as a friend. Abu Hassan had warned Khalid about people who wanted to hurt him. The jinn had even convinced Khalid to turn away from the neo-orthodox Muslims in the mosque where I worked, claiming that their practice of Islam was degenerated and corrupt. At a certain point, however, Khalid realised that the jinn possessing him was in fact the same jinn who had previously possessed his older brother before he committed suicide. Indeed he found out that the form of Islam Abu Hassan had convinced him to follow was a forgery, and that the real purpose of the jinn was to drive him towards the same ill-fated destination as his deceased brother. Khalid was left in a religious vacuum, having rejected his previous faith practices in the neo-orthodox mosques and then discovering that his current practices were simply the work of a jinn bent on driving him to suicide. He explained how he even had physical fights with Abu Hassan. The jinn would occupy a part of his body while he, from another part of the body, would try to fight back.

From an Islamic point of view, we could understand the stories of Abu Omar, Aziz, and Khalid as particular forms of idolatry in which the jinn disguises itself as divine law and then intrudes into the victims' interior through their attempts to fight evil by complying with certain rules. Indeed all of these possessed persons exhibited extreme obedience to a very strict interpretation of Islamic codes of conduct in the period leading up to their outbreaks. Perhaps we could even speculate that the jinn made them momentarily worship, not God, but these rules for their own sake. As several shaykhs made clear to me, this is by no means the intention with Islamic practices of worship. Prayer, fasting, almsgiving, and any other work of faith is nothing in itself. Rather these practices are only to be understood as techniques for cultivating a pious self. Piety among other things consists of the ability of a person to feel humility (*khushūʿ*) and fear (*taqwā*). Strict attendance to the divine doctrine may be a necessary requirement for achieving such piety, but there is a way in which strict attendance to the rules may also result in arrogance (*kibr*) and even self-righteousness – a risk that Abu Bilal also said was a danger in his work as an Islamic healer (see Chapter 6).

In a similar way, Anthony Steinbock (2007: 233) has pointed out how certain forms of fundamentalism can transform into illusions of self-mastery that excludes the possibility of religious experience, which for him is defined as the realisation of the form of 'givenness' that characterises human existence. I believe that in these microdynamics discussed by Abu Bilal and Steinbock we might find important clues for understanding not only how attempts to fight the jinn and eradicate evil can sometimes transform into the opposite, but also how the various attempts to 'map' Muslim communities, the ongoing securitisation of Danish society, and the so-called religious 'radicalisation' of certain Muslim communities have all resulted in an unfortunate escalation of fear and hatred over recent years (see Chapter 1; Suhr and Sinclair 2016).

What would it be like to live with a husband taken over by an overzealous adherence to, even veneration of, strict religious rules? How should I understand Umm Omar's keen efforts to make me film her husband's exorcism in the best way possible? In contrast to my handheld close-ups and half totals, constantly moving in and out of proper perspectival distance, the body as seen from up there on that tripod could have been contemplated and contained within the frame of the image. It would not so excessively have exploded the frame of the image. It might in fact have been the exact 'optimal distance' from where to grasp this body of aggression and pain (Willerslev 2009a). Umm Omar was not the one possessed by a spirit, but she was still subjected to the jinn that possessed her husband. Perhaps it was an attempt to show the form of madness she was subjected to in her marriage. Perhaps it was even a form of resistance – a way of providing a testimony of her situation, and of showing the way she attempted to handle it. Such conclusions might in a roundabout way have brought us closer towards the framework of scholars such as Boddy (1989), El-Kholy (2002), and Rothenberg (2004), who locate in spirit possession a possibility for semi-autonomous, female, and counter-hegemonic agency in a mad world characterised by sexist and post-colonial oppression.

In this book I have preferred to stay on the outside of the explanations given by people of their own suffering and the healing practices they engage in. In doing so I have paid special attention to resistance, mainly in the sense of *ṣabr*, the capacity of humans to remain hopeful and to endure the hardships of life. But the struggle of the self is also to oppose oppression, such as occurs with the unlawful intrusion of evil expressed in jinn possession. The Islamic practice of *ruqya* may facilitate the cultivation of patience, and the recitation of multiple verses from the Quran may expose both the jinn and human subject to the frailty of earthly existence. Yet at the same time *ruqya* is clearly also aimed at ending the illegal occupation of the jinn, so that the human subject may repossess its body. Umm Omar was pointing towards a more direct mode of witnessing her and her husband's situation. Perhaps she was also pointing to a more active stance of resistance, than what I have been able to convey through the film and describe in this book.

## Beyond the time-image

The third puzzle I wish to address here concerns Deleuze's account of the evolution of modern cinema. In Deleuze's theory of film, we end up with the establishment of the time-image – an image allowing viewers the possibility of becoming witnesses and seers. For Deleuze, the promise of the time-image is the reinstatement of belief in the world. As he writes, modern cinema makes us 'believe, not in a different world, but in a link between man and the world, in love or life, to believe in this as in the impossible, the unthinkable, which nonetheless cannot but be thought' (Deleuze 2005b: 164). Even though Deleuze locates this development in the rise of a particular form of avant-garde cinema in the mid-twentieth century, many of his formulations resonate well with Kierkegaard's understanding of the double movement of faith conceived of as the resignation from the world and the taking it up again on the strength of the absurd (Deleuze 2005b: 171; Kierkegaard 2005: 45).

In Chapter 6 I discussed how particular forms of disruptive montage can be applied to understand how psychiatric consultations and Islamic exorcisms both work to dismantle the illusion of autonomous human agency, and thereby facilitate the possibility of a leap of faith. The idea of understanding the Quran and the ritual practices of worship among my interlocutors through the prism of cinema began in 2009 after a discussion with Said, a young Somali university student. In response to my regret about feeling unable to read the Quran, finding it too difficult and complex, Said referred me to a YouTube lecture about the 'Literary Characteristics of the Quran' by Nouman Ali Khan (2009). Here the divine speech was made sense of by attributing to it the aesthetics of the modern medium of film. Hirschkind (2006: 155) performs a similar operation in an analysis of the cinematic qualities in Islamic cassette sermons in Cairo. One way of understanding this coupling between a modern medium of expression and religious practices of worship would be to see it as an effort to reconsolidate religious practices within the modern secular era – a popularisation and modernisation of Islam in order to make it attractive to a new type of religious consumer. Yet there are other ways of looking at it. As described in Chapter 6, Kapferer (2013) and Marks (2010) take a very different view of the relationship between religious art, ritual aesthetics, and modern media. As Kapferer points out, ritual always had the 'cinematic' qualities we now find in modern cinema.

Taking the cue from Said as well as Kapferer, Marks, and Khan, I have explored the ritual use of 'cinematic' forms in psychiatric and Islamic treatments. Nevertheless there are obvious differences between cinema and ritual I have still not adequately addressed. In ritual, access to the 'cinematic' mode of perception is mediated in 'real-time' by the healer or ritual specialist. This means that contrary to the frozen form of a film, the ritual is able to adjust itself according to the immediate requirements of the concrete situation.

Video and audio recordings of *ruqya* and Quranic recitations abound and are freely available to view and download online. Even though playing these may have devotional effects, as we saw in the consumption of neo-orthodox YouTube exorcisms (see Chapter 3 and Scene 7), they are not, however, sufficiently powerful to expel a jinn from a human body. To perform such an operation, a mediation needs to take place by which a ritual specialist conveys the power of the divine words to the patient in ways specifically designed to be in line with their problems.

As Jørgen Aagaard argues regarding psychiatric healthcare, it is the procedures by which a medication is provided to a patient that counts for the most (Scene 11). Medication, whether in the form of Islamic recitations or psychotropics, apparently has to be invested personally in particular settings. As Abu Bilal argues, Quranic recitations achieve their full power only when they are recited with pure intention and ask God for healing to be released at a particular moment in time and space. We could perhaps say that the cinematic qualities Deleuze associates with modern film can be even better and more powerfully expressed in a real-time live ritual. This uniqueness inherent in particular healing interventions of the divine or psychotropics – what in Benjamin's (1968: 221–3) terms would be associated with 'aura' – is often lost in the frozen form of modern cinema.

If we agree with Kapferer in his joining of ritual to cinema, we must add that the cinematic aesthetics he describes seem more efficient and powerful in 'live, real-time' ritual than in actual film. Or to put it in other words: film is a weak replication of the 'cinematic' qualities inherent to certain forms of ritual. While my recordings of exorcisms and psychiatric consultations display an enormous amount of visible detail, the absent-presence of the invisible, God, or 'the view from everywhere' is never really evoked as it is in 'live' ritual. Sometimes, after a severe re-edit, this peculiar auratic presence reappears, but only to disappear after one or two additional screenings. Indeed, as Hastrup observed with regard to her Icelandic ram photography, it appears as if the images provided by modern cameras very easily become flat. I have come to conclude that the power of these healing rituals simply cannot be captured in a fixed visual form. As Merleau-Ponty and Marion would put it, such power can only be evoked through its absence. This is perhaps why iconoclasm has become all the more important in the age of mechanical reproduction (see also Adorno 1984: 223). To attain the aura of ritual, cinema needs to provide an authentic shock – a shock that cannot be replicated, but has to be continuously developed and replaced by new forms and aesthetic techniques.

The shaping of the film and book has been inspired by the cinematic montage proposed by early Soviet filmmakers such as Eisenstein and Vertov, as well as by Deleuze's film theory. As a whole, the film and book might even seem to parallel the disruptive movements of psychiatric and Islamic treatments that I have analysed with reference to these filmmakers and theorists, as well as Kierkegaard's double movement of faith. While many of the scenes are still rather lengthy, I have attempted to cut them in a way that does not tame the interactions between healers and patients in terms of cultural stereotypes or narrative plots. One might say that the film becomes almost non-anthropological in its disregard for standard sociological schemes of interpretation. Suspending narrative plots and sociological schemes allows the film to evoke the ways in which both psychiatric and Islamic treatments often discount the narratives of patients as sufficient explanations of their condition in favour of agencies external to the world of humans. But what kind of world arises on the other side of the time-image or the double movement of faith? In what sense can we talk about these movements as a mode of healing?

In Deleuze, what is of utmost political importance is the way the time-image gives rise to a sort of unbounded becoming of new subjectivities. This vision of pure becoming is centred around his idea of modern cinema as a generator of 'free, indirect discourse and vision' (Deleuze 2005b: 144). In addition to pioneering filmmakers such as Orson Welles, Jean-Luc Godard, Stanley Kubrick, and Werner Herzog, Deleuze also makes mention of one of the founding fathers of ethnographic filmmaking, namely Jean Rouch (see Chapters 1 and 3). What emerged with Rouch's collaborative way of producing ethnofictions in companionship with his field interlocutors was, in Deleuze's view, the establishment of a form of subjectivity that was neither Rouch's nor that of the people in his films. Discussing *Jaguar* (Rouch 1967) and the widely debated *Les Maîtres Fous* (Rouch 1955) about a *hauka* spirit-possession cult in Ghana during the last days of British colonial rule, Deleuze (2005b: 148) argues that these films constitute the documentation of an 'I' always in the process of becoming 'another'.

Special attention is also paid to Rouch's films in Taussig's (1993) work on the mimetic faculty. For Taussig, the *hauka* cult of *Les Maîtres Fous* appears as a parodic form of resistance to and subversion of imperial power. This interpretation is evoked by Rouch's juxtaposition of a shot featuring *hauka* performers cracking an egg on the head of a statue – presumably representing the British governor – with a shot of the real governor wearing a white plumed helmet (Taussig 1993: 243; see also Russell 1999: 224). From such examples, Taussig comes to the optimistic conclusion that in the paradoxical mimicry made visible through Rouch's montage, colonial – and by extension anthropological – mastery is no longer possible: 'What remains is unsettled and unsettling interpretation in constant movement with itself … because the interpreting self is itself grafted into the object of study. The self enters into the alter against which the self is defined and sustained' (Taussig 1993: 237).

For Taussig, a zone of vacuity or 'imageric possibility' – what I have here called the invisible ground of alterity – arises when self and other, in 'ordered disorder' and 'continuous discontinuity', are turned upside down and made strange. As Taussig puts it, montage is a manner of 'interruptedness' – a device for provoking 'sudden and infinite connections between dissimilars in an endless or almost endless process of connection-making and connection-breaking … which on account of its awkwardness of fit, cracks, and violent juxtapositionings can actively embody both a presentation and a counter-presentation' (1986: 441–3).

In this analysis I have described how montage, as a manner of 'interruptedness', and the time-image, as proposed by Deleuze, may be useful for understanding the dissolution of self occurring in Danish psychiatry and Islamic exorcisms. But what happens beyond the time-images that are established in these particular ethnographic settings? Certainly it is a matter of emancipation from the oppression and tyranny of the illnesses causing the suffering of patients. Nevertheless, to understand the outcome of the dissolution of subjectivity and human agency as the emergence of a 'free indirect discourse and vision' might be too optimistic.

For Deleuze as well as Taussig, disruptive montage enables a setting free of human creativity from its enslavement and subordination to fixed, doctrinal subject positions. In this, both Taussig and Deleuze clearly depart from the early Hegel's idea that human freedom is only possible through realisation of one's inevitable dispossession and enslavement. Instead they take a step towards Friedrich Nietzche's Dionysian rebirth of the subject in the figure of the *Übermensch*. Not anti-humanism, but a kind of super-humanism should be the correct term to describe this particular form of subjectivity releasing itself so completely from the oppressive 'slave moral' of politico-religious ideologies and instead becoming what Deleuze (2005b: 150) refers to as 'we, creators of truth' (see also Kapferer 2014).

But as indicated in Chapters 3 and 6, beyond the time-image could also lie, not just the liberated avant-garde artist, but the establishment of a new order – an order flowing from within what Deleuze would call the realm of the 'virtual' and what the people I worked with would call God or modern biomedicine (Benjamin 1968: 234; Schwartz 2005). In these settings the aim of the time-image is to produce a life that flows from within the liminal sphere of ritual. For my informants, the value of the Quran, as a particular kind of 'time-image' that testifies to the presence of an omnipresent and all-powerful God throughout space and time, is not to set free human discourse, but rather its capacity to allow human life to be reassumed from within the space of ritual, that is, to be structured entirely by the divine, thereby installing in earthly life a preliminary taste of paradise – a momentary flowing without obstacles and tension. Kapferer (2013) also points out how the time-image in the Sinhala anti-sorcery rituals in Sri Lanka works in this way: not to release the subject to free-floating artistic becoming, but to reinstall the subject according to the laws of the cosmos.

So what could the nature of this all-encompassing structuring power be that patients undergoing psychiatric healthcare and Islamic exorcism need to submit to in order to resume a life worth living? My hunch is that it is quite far from Deleuze's attractive Dionysian idea of 'love' and 'life'. Nor is it a kind of altruistic, non-violent, non-deterministic being with others. Rather, I think we need to reconsider that long-despised, rational, maximising drive for self-interest most clearly depicted in the notion of 'homo economicus'.

Surely the economic pursuit of self-interest must be a key element of any capitalist system, but in many ways capitalisation is also found in Islamic practices of worship. Thus it was often emphasised to me how the only sphere of life where competition is relevant and worthwhile is religion: one should do everything in one's powers to maximise one's prospects for a good place in the afterlife. Thus it is said that a Friday prayer performed by a man in the mosque will be rewarded with twenty-seven times as many blessings (*ḥasanāt*) compared to if he had done the prayer at home. Furthermore, additional blessings are added if one has a long way to walk to the mosque and if one stands first in the prayer row. Quite meticulous systems for counting the number of blessings were also related to me with regard to the voluntary supplications (*du'ā'*) and remembrance of God (*dhikr*) performed after or between prayers, and for performing prayers during the shift of the angels in the time before daybreak. Even more rewarding are the supplications performed by people suffering from illness.

Most rewarding of all prayers is the prayer towards the end of Ramadan during Laylat al-Qadr (the night of glory or destiny). On this particular night it is said that vast numbers of angels descend to earth, providing an exceptional opportunity for prayers to be heard. According to the Quran (Surat al-Qadr 1–5) and the hadith, this special prayer is better than a thousand months, equivalent, that is, to a whole lifetime of constant worship. As described in Chapter 5, Islamic practices of faith such as these can be seen as a form of self-sacrifice that is at once a gesture of unconditional commitment to the divine, as well as an instrumental act of offering one's work in the hope of greater profit in the afterlife. All of these practices trying to amass the blessings of God have the ultimate aim of establishing the possibility of being close to God and of ensuring the most pleasurable situation for oneself in the afterlife.

In a roundabout way, the urge towards pursuing and maximising individual self-interest in both psychiatric healthcare and neo-orthodox Islam seems to be directed towards exactly the kind of economic thinking that has also been posited as the driving engine in many anthropological theories of practice (see e.g. Bourdieu 1977; Ortner 1984; Barth 1987). In fact this is also how Kierkegaard imagines the knight of faith. In his essay he describes the knight not as a poet, virtuoso artist, or militant hero, but as the epitome of an ordinary person who meticulously attends to the needs and requirements of everyday life:

> Here he is ... Good God! Is this the person, is it really him? He looks just like a tax-gatherer ... you would think he was some pen-pusher who had lost his soul to Italian book-keeping ... a shop-keeper ... a postman ... a *restaurateur*. (Kierkegaard 2005: 42–3, italics in the original)

Freud too asserted an economic drive at the root of a normal well-functioning psyche. As he states:

> In psychoanalytic theory we assume without further ado that the evolution of psychic processes is automatically regulated by the pleasure principle; that is to say, we believe that these processes are invariably triggered by an unpleasureable tension, and then follow a path such that their ultimate outcome represents a diminution of this tension, and hence a propensity to avoid unpleasure or to generate pleasure. (Freud 2003: 45)

While Freud describes the operation of the pleasure principle within a purely secular and 'worldly' ontology, he also identifies how the drive towards maximum pleasure at the deepest stratum of analysis is a drive towards the kind of stability that can only be obtained in death. Since nothing in earthly life can be pure pleasure, Freud posits the 'reality principle' as the sensible psychic mechanics, the economic effort of Kierkegaard's Italian bookkeeper, that seeks not to eliminate pleasure, but to postpone it so that it is not disappointed and turned into disillusion or aggression. The overarching aim of life in Freud's model of the human psyche is thus to release and return itself back to an inorganic state, the ultimate pleasure of death, in the most economic and 'natural' way.

If we can say that the ideal endpoint of psychiatric healthcare is to restore the subject to the possibility of taking its place as both producer and consumer in the capitalist economy, the ultimate aim of neo-orthodox Islamic worship is the accumulation of blessings that will facilitate access to the boundless pleasures of paradise. Rather than how to overcome the economic principle operating within the human mind, the question for psychoanalysis, as for Danish psychiatric healthcare, neo-orthodox Islam, and Kierkegaard, is therefore how to accept the existence of this principle and channel it towards the best possible destination.

However, as Freud pointed out, economic thinking may easily transform into a brutal and destructive drive. Often the pleasure principle can 'lead astray' and be transformed into a predatory consumption and corruption of life (see Pandolfo 2007: 350–1). We could perhaps see this happening when the subject of psychiatric healthcare is not returned as a contributor to the capitalist market, but instead becomes encapsulated and entrapped within an ever-increasing spiral of psychotropic medication. In these cases, psychiatry appears not to be a form of healing, but rather the effect of an excessive human engineering gone wild. Perhaps we could also see this happening when, in neo-orthodox Islam, worship sometimes appears to become derailed and transformed into a cultivation of self-righteousness rather than humility. It seems that these dangers have to be taken seriously when considering both systems of treatment.

In this project I have been inspired by the disruptive principle of montage, a principle which may also be seen at work in the treatments of both psychiatric healthcare and Islamic exorcism. In both these treatments, disruption should ideally lead to a reassemblage, a return of the patient towards some form of stability. Yet there is a constant danger that these treatments may deteriorate into forms of idolatrous self-righteousness, or human engineering, that are far removed from the modest economic bookkeeper and tax-gatherer described by Kierkegaard. Perhaps something similar can be said about the use of montage as a disruptive principle for anthropological writing and filmmaking.

In a thought-provoking article, Paul Henley (2006: 40) re-evaluates Rouch's classic film about the *hauka* spirit possession cult and points out that what goes on in the actual observational scene cannot be simply reduced to a parodic subversion of colonial mastery, as proposed by both Taussig and Deleuze. Instead Henley (2006: 754–6) finds sufficient evidence in the film footage and in ethnographic descriptions of spirit possession in West Africa to suggest that, rather than an example of counter-hegemonic resistance, the cultic event is a fertility ritual, modelled on the North African *zār* cult, where ritual participants attempt to assimilate the power of influential figures for religious purposes. The colonial mockery suggested by Rouch's montage, which in Deleuze and Taussig's view worked to evoke the subversive alterity of spirit possession, is in Henley's re-evaluation better understood as an attempt to make the possession ritual acceptable to the political preferences of anthropologists and African intellectuals in Paris (Henley 2006: 37).

We may take Henley's example as a reminder against quick assumptions of montage as being somehow intrinsically emancipative. The subversive potential of montage lies in its capacity for altering the obvious perception of an object, image, or perspective by combining two or more elements. As Benjamin argued, montage thereby facilitates a 'denaturalization', which may convey just how deeply questionable that which we tend to take as reality actually is (Buck-Morss 1991: 71, 218). Yet montage is not only an amplifier of invisibility and instability. As made clear also in Chapter 3, montage is the splintering of pre-established orders of visuality, but is also its reassembling (Benjamin 1968: 234).

This book has been an attempt to appreciate the work of the invisible as an unknowable ground of human existence. With the neo-orthodox Islamic resistance to visualising the invisible (*al-ghayb*), as well as with writers such as Levinas and Merleau-Ponty, I have suggested that there may be important ethical and epistemological reasons within the discipline of anthropology for keeping the invisible invisible. Yet, as with the discussion of doubt and resistance above, there may be a tipping point. There may be a situation where the urge not to completely visualise the alterity of the other convolutes into an aesthetics that could create a fetish of the invisible and the unknown, even in situations where there really is a lot to see and know, and a lot which should be seen and known – such as, for example, when madness becomes so coercive that it assumes a visible form that can be seen and calls for resistance and action.

Just as the colonising operation of vision and the ocularcentric tendency of much social science may do immense harm to the alterity of others as well as the perceiving self, so might a denial of vision preclude the possibility of witnessing things that should be seen, and foreclose the possibility of discourse where things should be said (see e.g. MacDougall 2006: 8; Kreinath 2012: 296–7). Henley points to the dangers of montage in his analysis of *Les Maîtres Fous*, a film highlighted by both Taussig and Deleuze as the coming into being of free-floating human creativity, but which Henley shows us could also be interpreted as an elimination of the alterity of a spirit possession cult. Perhaps Umm Omar was also, like Henley, asserting the value of cinematic realism and photographic documentation as sometimes being a more powerful standpoint for resistance to oppression than the fragmented and fragmentary techniques of montage. Ethnographic filmmaking and montage is an almost impossible yet necessary balancing act that occurs along this stretch between the visible and the invisible, the expressible and inexpressible; between witnessing those things that should be seen, disrupting the ways in which we have been taught to see, while at the same time allowing a space for that which cannot be seen.

## The magic in Feisal

If these last 'Aleph'-like figures that continue to stick in my mind point towards the value of ethnographic realism, the importance of resistance, and perhaps even a 'moderate' form of humanism, I wish to finish this book by returning to the people whose continuous struggles make any resort to quick analytic conclusions difficult. Most of the people we have met in the previous pages never really seemed to achieve healing as such. Rather their encounters with psychiatric healthcare and Islamic exorcism seem to be part of an ongoing attempt to cope with the hardships of life.

Abu Hassan, the jinn who had possessed Khalid (see Chapter 5), as well as the jinn of Abdel Rahman's brother (see Chapter 4), seem to continue their damaging work. At times they disappear for a while, only to return again with an equally destructive force. After a number of additional exorcisms Abu Omar eventually did seem to get rid of the jinn and the magic that had haunted him for years, but he is still struggling with other things in his life. Nadia, whom we met in Chapter 4, is in a similar situation. After Abu Bilal recommended she take down the photos in her room, she was relieved of her nightmares (see Chapter 6), but after a trip to Bosnia the following year she suffered a relapse. She recovered again but recently her mother entered a state of depression, possibly due to the same source of magic that caused her daughter's problems.

A similar pattern of continuous struggle seems to apply to the psychiatric patients I followed. In autumn 2011 it seemed as if Aziz had finally accepted psychiatric treatment, and indeed he appeared more stable than I had ever seen him before. But during Ramadan the following year he suffered a major relapse. According to him, this was the third time the jinn had returned. Every second year the magic seems to be reactivated, and it always seems to happen towards the end of Ramadan. Esther was not surprised that these outbreaks occurred during the fasting of Ramadan since, as she points out, the inversion of the natural sleep rhythm is itself a symptom of psychosis.

Aziz was immediately returned to the psychiatric hospital. This time, however, he was transferred to the department of forensic psychiatry and an entirely new set of psychiatrists and nurses. The psychiatrists re-diagnosed his condition as bipolar disorder. This disorder would seem to be significantly milder than Aziz's previous diagnosis of paranoid schizophrenia, but nevertheless the psychiatrists decided to increase his medication by adding the anti-epileptic drug Delepsine. He was still prescribed Zyprexa (olanzapine), but now the psychiatrists decided to administer the drug through intra-muscular injection as they suspected he had not taken all the tablets he had been prescribed.

According to Aziz, he was being accused of criminal activities. One psychiatrist had apparently told him that the next time he had a psychotic relapse he would be hospitalised for the rest of his life. At the beginning of Aziz's hospitalisation, some quarrels occurred between people who wanted to visit Aziz and the hospital staff. It was therefore decided that Aziz could not receive any visitors other than his wife, children, and his anthropologist.

Not even Aziz's shaykh was allowed access to the hospital. Quite obviously, Aziz was in great distress when I visited him.

Since then Aziz has been in and out of hospital a number of times. We are in contact on a regular basis. He uses the film we made to explain his situation to the hospital staff and to his friends. The staff now allows visits by his shaykh if he requests them, but despite numerous Quranic and psychiatric treatments, the jinn, the magic, and the side effects of Zyprexa and Delepsine still cause him a lot of pain.

Feisal's situation is also complicated. After a number of exorcisms, Abu Bilal and Feisal eventually agreed that he needed treatment by a more experienced shaykh. Abu Bilal contacted and set up a meeting with a well-regarded scholar of Islamic *ʿaqīda* who lives in a southern suburb of Aarhus. This shaykh had a different and more definitive take on the performance of *ruqya* than Abu Bilal. Feisal was asked to sit on his knees in front of a sofa. A friend of Feisal and I were asked to sit on the sides. Abu Bilal and the other shaykh sat on the sofa, facing Feisal.

The shaykh began the exorcism by placing his right hand on Feisal's head and reciting the Quran into Feisal's right ear. Yet in contrast to Abu Bilal's recitation, the voice of the shaykh was both louder and more aggressive in tone. Furthermore it was oriented directly into the ear, with only a few centimetres between his mouth and Feisal's head. The jinn almost immediately emerged in Feisal, screaming and shouting in pain. It was a monotonous recitation; more like the sound of a drone than the melodious recitation of Abu Bilal. It continued almost without any changes in volume or pace. At times the jinn tried to say something to the shaykh, but he just continued his recitation, ignoring any attempts of the jinn to enter into a dialogue. A few times, Abu Bilal, on the sofa next to the shaykh, would remind him that the jinn was trying to speak. The shaykh continued to torment the jinn, completely absorbed in his attempt to eradicate its presence from Feisal's body.

As the exorcism proceeded, it became very uncomfortable for me to witness and be a part of. I had to leave the room. I am not sure how much time passed, but it was by far the longest exorcism I have attended. It was released not in the form of crying, as had happened on previous occasions with Feisal. Instead it seemed as if the resistant energy in Feisal just gradually departed. After the exorcism, he was completely exhausted. His knees had gone to sleep from sitting in this position for such a long time. I for my part had had enough. This was beyond what I could cope with.

In the days after the exorcism, Feisal claimed he felt better. He decided to attend yet another exorcism with this shaykh. I could not attend. I was worried that the *ruqya* was getting out of hand and that this form of aggression might just as well inflict a serious psychosis or traumatisation as remove a jinn. I realised that I had reached the limits of my capacity for belief. As much as I had attempted to take seriously Abu Bilal's understanding of the mechanisms at work in the expelling of jinn, I realised that this had been too easy for me, since Abu Bilal's compassionate and empathic way of reciting the Quran had never directly opposed my previous view of the world. As Esther remarked, his voice was of such a beauty that it surely had to be a healing one way or another. I discovered that all along, I had been able to attribute the agentive capacity of healing not to the power of the divine words, but to Abu Bilal's skills as a virtuoso in the art of Quranic recitation. Indeed I found myself caught in exactly the form of humanism that I was intellectually trying to argue against.

During those days I tried to make both Feisal, his friend, and Abu Bilal understand the possible dangers that could be inflicted by a serious traumatisation of the psyche. They still insisted that Feisal was benefiting from the exorcism and that he should have further treatments. After one exorcism, which lasted several hours, Abu Bilal came to show me a video he had made with his iPhone. He wanted me to see the real power of *ruqya*. Feisal had allowed him to show me the video but insisted on it being deleted afterwards. In the video Feisal was seen lying on the white carpet of his living room, behind the sofa. His arms and legs were spread to both sides as if he had been dropped to the floor from above. His head was bent to the side. From his mouth and all around him there was blood, vomit, and clots of a dark substance which Abu Bilal told me was magic. Stains of blood had also hit the wall.

I have seen other patients vomiting during exorcisms, but not to this extent. Feisal was breathing, though. Abu Bilal made it clear the shaykh had not hit him or physically forced him to vomit. The magic had simply left Feisal due to the recitation of the Quran.

I called Feisal. He told me his stomach was hurting, but that in his mind he felt a great relief. I was dumbfounded. A few days later I had to leave Denmark for a six-month stay at the University of California in Berkeley. I had planned this stay for some time, and it was not only to study. As fieldwork had led me deeper into Islamic practices of worship, I had felt an increasing urge to flee and escape it all. Whilst at Berkeley I heard the exorcisms of Feisal continued and that even more magic had been ejected, along with blood and vomit. I was worried about the day Abu Bilal would call and tell me Feisal's jinn had finally succeeded in making him commit suicide.

When I returned to Denmark six months later, Feisal was in an entirely different shape than when I left him. His hair was cut and combed backward with a generous amount of gel. His clothes were respectable. His skin seemed to have gained a bit of colour. His eyes were sharper, more focused and steadfast than I remembered them. He claimed the exorcisms had made a difference. Every now and then he still felt as though someone was sticking knives into his leg, but the voices demanding he kill himself had stopped.

I still have not made up my mind about the story of Feisal. He certainly looked significantly better when I returned to Denmark. Somehow he is living visible proof of the efficacy of an extreme form of Quranic recitation, whose healing power lies far beyond what I could possibly explain in any standard academic vocabulary. Yet I am worried that at some point all these invisible spirits will return and he will be back where he was before. He claims he is much better, and this is the important thing. Now Feisal's main problem is that some of his jinn seem to have resettled in the lower leg of his wife, Sara. Lately Sara has started behaving in odd ways which – according to Feisal – cannot but be interpreted as possession by jinn. He tells me she doesn't agree, however. Rejecting jinn possession as the cause of her problems, she went to her physician and is now being treated for epilepsy; the condition which in its Arabic translation – *ṣarʿ* – marks the descent of consciousness into invisibility.

# References

## Books and articles


Aagaard, Jørgen, Lars Merinder, and Dorthe Mundbjerg. 2009. Psykoedukation. In *Psykiatrisk Sygepleje*. Niels Buus, ed. Pp. 364–82. Copenhagen: Dansk Sygeplejeråd and Nyt Nordisk Forlag Arnold Busck.

Abu-Lughod, Lila. 1986. *Veiled Sentiments: Honor and Poetry in a Bedouin Society*. Berkeley: University of California Press.

Adorno, Theodor W. 1984. *Aesthetic Theory*. C. Lenhardt, trans. London and Boston: Routledge and Kegan Paul.

Al-Ghazali, Abu Hamid Muhammad. 1989[1058–1111 C.E.]. *The Remembrance of Death and the Afterlife*. T. Winter, trans. Cambridge: Islamic Texts Society.

Al-Issa, Ihsan. 2000. Preface. In *Al-Junūn: Mental Illness in the Islamic World*. Ihsan Al-Issa, ed. Pp. xiii–xv. Madison: International Universities Press.

Al-Jawziyah, Ibn Qayyim. 2003[1292–1350 C.E.]. *Healing with the Medicine of the Prophet*. Abdul Rahman Abdullah, ed. Jalal Abual Rub, trans. Riyadh: Darussalam.

Altorki, Soraya. 1986. *Women in Saudi Arabia: Ideology and Behavior among the Elite*. New York: Columbia University Press.

Anderson, Benedict. 1991. *Imagined Communities: Reflections on the Origin and Spread of Nationalism*. New York: Verso Books.

Arnheim, Rudolf. 1957. *Film as Art*. Berkeley: University of California Press.

Asad, Talal. 2003. *Formations of the Secular: Christianity, Islam, Modernity*. Stanford: Stanford University Press.

Axinn, Sidney. 2010. *Sacrifice and Value: A Kantian Interpretation*. Lanham and Plymouth: Lexington Books.

Badeen, Edward and Birgit Krawietz. 2003. Islamic Reinvention of Jinn: Status-Cut and Success Story. In *Identidades Marginales*. Cristina de la Puente, ed. Pp. 93–109. Madrid: Consejo Superior de Investigaciones Cientificas.

Baker, C. Bruce, Michael Johnsrud, Lynn Crismon, Robert Rosenheck, and Scott Woods. 2003. Quantitative Analysis of Sponsorship Bias in Economic Studies of Antidepressants. *The British Journal of Psychiatry* 183(6): 498–506.

Bankovsky, Miriam. 2004. A Thread of Knots: Jacques Derrida's Homage to Emmanuel Levinas's Ethical Reminder. *Invisible Culture* 8: 1–19.

Barker, Phil and Poppy Buchanan-Barker. 2009. En Søgen efter Personen: Tidal-Modellen og Holistisk Assessment. In *Psykiatrisk Sygepleje*. Niels Buus, ed. Copenhagen: Dansk Sygeplejeråd og Nyt Nordisk Forlag Arnold Busck.

Barnes, John A. 1987. Edward Evan Evans-Pritchard, 1902–1973. *Proceedings of the British Academy* LXXIII: 447–90.

Barth, Fredrik. 1966. *Models of Social Organization*. London: Royal Anthropological Institute.

———. 1987. *Cosmologies in the Making: A Generative Approach to Cultural Variation in Inner New Guinea*. Cambridge: Cambridge University Press.

Barthes, Roland. 2010[1980]. *Camera Lucida: Reflections on Photography*. Richard Howard, trans. New York: Farrar, Straus and Giroux.

Basso, Elisabetta. 2011. Maurice Merleau-Ponty: Kierkegaard's Influence on His Work. *Kierkegaard and Existentialism* 9: 233–61.

Bataille, George. 1991[1967]. *The Accursed Share: Volume 1: Consumption*. Robert Hurley, trans. New York: Zone Books.

Bazin, André. 2005[1967]. *What is Cinema? Volume 1*. Hugh Gray, trans. Berkeley: University of California Press.

BBC News. 2012. Naila Mumtaz Murder: Four Family Members Jailed For Life. Newspaper article. Retrieved 11 October 2018. www.bbc.co.uk/news/uk-england-birmingham-19699500

Behrend, Heike, Anja Dreschke, and Martin Zillinger, eds. 2015. *Trance Mediums and New Media: Spirit Possession in the Age of Technical Reproduction*. New York: Fordham University Press.

Bektovic, Safet. 1999. The Doubled Movement of Infinity in Kierkegaard and in Sufism. *Islam and Christian–Muslim Relations* 10: 325–37.

Benjamin, Walter. 1968. The Work of Art in the Age of Mechanical Reproduction. In *Illuminations*. Hannah Arendt, ed. and trans. Pp. 211–44. London: Fontana.

Berenson, Alex. 2007. Lilly Settles with 18,000 over Zyprexa. *New York Times*. Retrieved 8 March 2013. www.nytimes.com/2007/01/05/business/05drug.html?_r=0

Bille, Mikkel and Tim Flohr Sørensen. 2007. An Anthropology of Luminosity: The Agency of Light. *Journal of Material Culture* 12(3): 263–84.

Blanchot, Maurice. 1993[1969]. *The Infinite Conversation*. Susan Hanson, trans. Minneapolis: University of Minnesota Press.

Bloch, Maurice. 1992. *Prey into Hunter: The Politics of Religious Experience*. Cambridge: Cambridge University Press.

Bloom, Floyd E. 2010. Placebo Versus Antidepressant Review: The Emperor's New Drugs: Exploding the Antidepressant Myth. *Cerebrum*. Retrieved 8 March 2013. http://dana.org/news/cerebrum/detail.aspx?id=28024

Boddy, Janice. 1989. *Wombs and Alien Spirits: Women, Men, and the Zār Cult in Northern Sudan*. Madison: The University of Wisconsin Press.

———. 1994. Spirit Possession Revisited: Beyond Instrumentality. *Annual Review of Anthropology* 23: 407–34.

Boe, Carolina Sanchez. 2017. From Jyllands-Posten to Charlie Hebdo: Domesticating The Muhamed Cartoons. In *Suis-je Charlie? Politics and Media after the Paris Attacks*. Gavan Titley, Des Freedman, Gholam Khiabany, and Aurélien Mondon, eds. London: Zed Books.

Boe, Carolina Sanchez and Peter Hervik. 2008. Integration through Insult. In *Transnational Media Events. The Mohammed Cartoons and the Imagined Clash of Civilizations*. Elizabeth Eide, Risto Kunelius, and Angela Phillips, eds. Pp. 213–34. Nordicom: Gothenburg.

Borberg, Hjarn v. Zernichow. 2016. *Nydansk: Er nydanskere og danskere virkelig så forskellige?* Copenhagen: Multivers.

Borges, Jorge L. 1971. *The Aleph and Other Stories 1933–1969: Together with Commentaries and an Autobiographical Essay*. Norman Thomas di Giovanni, ed. and trans. London: Jonathan Cape.

Boseley, Sarah. 2018. The Drugs Do Work: Antidepressants Are Effective, Study Shows. *The Guardian*. 21 February 2018. Retrieved 15 January 2019. www.theguardian.com/science/2018/feb/21/the-drugs-do-work-antidepressants-are-effective-study-shows

Bourdieu, Pierre. 1977. *Outline of a Theory of Practice*. Cambridge: Cambridge University Press.

Breggin, Peter. 2008. *Brain Disabling Treatments in Psychiatry: Drugs, Electroshock, and the Psychopharmaceutical Complex*. New York: Springer Publishing Company.

Bruns, Gerald A. 2006. The Concepts of Art and Poetry in Emmanuel Levinas's Writings. In *The Cambridge Companion to Levinas*. Simon Critchley and Robert Bernasconi, eds. Pp. 206–33. Cambridge: Cambridge University Press.

Bubandt, Nils. 2009. Interview with an Ancestor: Spirits as Informants and the Politics of Possession in North Maluku. *Ethnography* 10(3): 291–316.

———. 2014. *The Empty Seashell: Witchcraft and Doubt on an Indonesian Island*. Ithaca: Cornell University Press.

Bubandt, Nils, Mikkel Rytter, and Christian Suhr. 2017. A Second Look at Invisibility: Al-Ghayb, Islam, Ethnography. *Contemporary Islam*, e-publication ahead of print: 1–16.

Buck-Morss, Susan. 1991. *The Dialectics of Seeing: Walter Benjamin and the Arcades Project*. Cambridge, MA: MIT Press.

Callan, Alyson. 2012. *Patients and Agents: Mental Illness, Modernity and Islam in Sylhet, Bangladesh*. New York: Berghahn Books.

Candea, Matei. 2011. Endo/Exo. *Common Knowledge* 17(1): 146–50.

Carter, Jeffrey. 2003. General Introduction. In *Understanding Religious Sacrifice: A Reader*. Jeffrey Carter, ed. Pp. 1–11. New York: Continuum.

Castaing-Taylor, Lucien. 1996. Iconophobia. *Transition* 69: 64–88.

Christensen, Mette Vedsgaard. 2003. Etnolekt i Århus Vest: Morfologiske, Syntaktiske og Pragmatiske Træk. In *Rapport fra MUDS 9*. Aarhus: Institut for Nordisk Sprog og Litteratur, Aarhus Universitet.

Cipriani, Andrea, Toshi A. Furukawa, Georgia Salanti, Anna Chaimani, Lauren Z. Atkinson, Yusuke Ogawa, Stefan Leucht, Henricus G. Ruhe, Erick H. Turner, Julian P. Higgins, Matthias Egger, Nozomi Takeshima, Yu Hayasaka, Hissei Imai, Kiyomi Shinohara, Aran Tajika, John P. A Loannidis, and John R. Geddes. 2018. Comparative Efficacy and Acceptability of 21 Antidepressant Drugs for the Acute Treatment of Adults with Major Depressive Disorder: A Systematic Review and Network Meta-analysis. *The Lancet*. 391(10128): 1357–66.

Clifford, James and George E. Marcus, eds. 1986. *Writing Culture: The Poetics and Politics of Ethnography*. Berkeley: University of California Press.

Connor, Linda, Timothy Asch, and Patsy Asch. 1986. *Jero Tapakan: Balinese Healer: An Etnographic Film Monograph*. Cambridge: Cambridge University Press.

Crapanzano, Vincent. 1973. *The Ḥamadsha: A Study in Moroccan Ethnopsychiatry*. Berkeley: University of California Press.

———. 1985. *Tuhami: Portrait of a Moroccan*. Chicago: University of Chicago Press.

Crapanzano, Vincent and Vivian Garrison, eds. 1977. *Case Studies in Spirit Possession*. New York: Wiley.

Csordas, Thomas. 1987. Health and the Holy in African and Afro-American Spirit Possession. *Social Science and Medicine* 24(1): 1–11.

———. 1990. Embodiment as a Paradigm for Anthropology. *Ethos* 18(1): 5–47.

———. 1997. *The Sacred Self: A Cultural Phenomenology of Charismatic Healing*. Berkeley: University of California Press.

Daily Mail. 2011. Muslim Mother Stabbed Daughter 40 Times and Cut Out Her Liver in Ritual Killing to 'Exorcise Evil Spirits'. Newspaper article. Retrieved 11 October 2018. www.dailymail.co.uk/news/article-2043813/Muslim-mother-stabbed-daughter-40-times-exorcise-evil-spirits-body.html

———. 2012. Muslim Woman 'Beaten with Walking Stick in Brutal Exorcism by Husband and Family who were Convinced She was Possessed by Demon'. Newspaper article. Retrieved 11 October 2018. www.dailymail.co.uk/news/article-2204968/Muslim-woman-beaten-walking-stick-brutal-exorcism-husband-family-members-convinced-possessed-demon.html

Danish Council of Ethics. 2012. Mødet med Patienten og Kulturen i Psykiatrien: Magt og Afmagt i Psykiatrien. Policy paper. Retrieved 15 January 2019. www.etiskraad.dk/~/media/Etisk-Raad/Etiske-Temaer/Psykiatri/Publikationer/2012-06-19-patienten-kulturen-psykiatrien.pdf

De Hert, Marc, Christoph U. Correll, and Dan Cohen. 2010. Do Antipsychotic Medications Reduce or Increase Mortality in Schizophrenia? A Critical Appraisal of the FIN-11 Study. *Schizophrenia Research* 117(1): 68–74.

Dein, Simon and Abdool Samad Illaiee. 2013. *Jinn* and Mental Health: Looking at *Jinn* Possession in Modern Psychiatric Practice. *The Psychiatrist Online* 37(9): 290–3.

Dein, Simon, Malcolm Alexander, and A. David Napier. 2008. *Jinn*, Psychiatry and Contested Notions of Misfortune among east London Bangladeshis. *Transcultural Psychiatry* 45(1): 31–55.

Deleuze, Gilles. 2005a[1986]. *Cinema 1: The Movement-Image*. Hugh Tomlinson and Barbara Habberjam, trans. London: Continuum.

———. 2005b[1989]. *Cinema 2: The Time-Image*. Hugh Tomlinson and Robert Galeta, trans. London: Continuum.

Dillon, Martin C. 1983. Merleau-Ponty and the Reversibility Thesis. *Man and World* 16(4): 365–88.

Doucet, Mathieu, and Sergio Sismondo. 2008. Evaluating Solutions to Sponsorship Bias. *Journal of Medical Ethics* 34(8): 627–30.

Douglas, Mary. 2002[1966]. *Purity and Danger: An Analysis of Concept of Pollution and Taboo*. London: Routledge.

Drachman, Hans, and Sebastian Goos. 2012. Psykisk Syge Dør Af Medicinen. Newspaper article. *Politiken*. Retrieved 7 March 2013. http://politiken.dk/indland/ECE1754922/psykisk-syge-doer-af-medicinen/

Drieskens, Barbara. 2008. *Living with Djinns: Understanding and Dealing with the Invisible in Cairo*. London: Saqi Books.

Durkheim, Émile. 2008[1912]. *The Elementary Forms of Religious Life*. Carol Cosman, trans. Oxford: Oxford University Press.

Edgerton, Robert B. 1971. A Traditional African Psychiatrist. *Southwestern Journal of Anthropology* 27(3): 259–78.

Eisenstein, Sergei M. 1949. *Film Form: Essays in Film Theory*. Jay Leyda, ed. and trans. New York: Harcourt Brace and Company.

———. 1988. *Selected Works*. Richard Taylor, ed. London: British Film Institute.

El-Kholy, Heba. 2002. *Defiance and Compliance: Negotiating Gender in Low-Income Cairo*. New York: Berghahn Books.

Elkins, James. 1996. *The Object Stares Back: On the Nature of Seeing*. New York: Simon & Schuster.

Esposito, John L. 1998. *Islam: The Straight Path*. New York: Oxford University Press.

Evans-Pritchard, E. E. 1956. *Nuer Religion*. Oxford: Clarendon Press.

———. 1965. *Theories of Primitive Religion*. Oxford: Oxford University Press.

———. 1970. Some Reflections on Mysticism. *DYN* 1: 99–116.

———. 1976[1937]. *Witchcraft, Oracles, and Magic among the Azande*. Oxford: Clarendon Press.

Fabian, Johannes. 2002. *Time and the Other: How Anthropology makes its Object*. New York: Columbia University Press.

Fadil, Nadia. 2011. Not-/Unveiling as an Ethical Practice. *Feminist Review* 98(1): 83–109.

Foucault, Michel. 1982. The Subject and Power. *Critical Inquiry* 8(4): 777–95.

———. 1988[1961]. *Madness and Civilization: A History of Insanity in the Age of Reason*. New York: Vintage Books.

———. 1997. On the Genealogy of Ethics: An Overview of Work in Progress. In *Ethics: Subjectivity and Truth. Essential Works of Foucault, 1954–1984, Vol 1*. Paul Rabinow, ed. Robert Hurley et al., trans. New York: New Press.

Fowler, W. W. 1920. The Original Meaning of the Word *Sacer*. In *Roman Essays and Interpretations*. Pp. 15–24. Oxford: Clarendon Press.

Fernando, Mayanthi L. 2010. Reconfiguring Freedom: Muslim Piety and the Limits of Secular Law and Public Discourse in France. *American Ethnologist* 37(1): 19–35.

———. 2014. *The Republic Unsettled: Muslim French and the Contradictions of Secularism*. Durham, NC: Duke University Press.

Freud, Sigmund. 1959[1912]. The Dynamics of Transference. In *Collected Papers of Sigmund Freud Volume 2*. Joan Riviere, ed. and trans. Pp. 323–41. New York: Basic Books.

———. 1980[1899]. *The Interpretation of Dreams*. New York: Avon.

———. 1989[1933]. *New Introductory Lectures on Psycho-analysis*. London: W. W. Norton & Company.

———. 2001[1917]. Mourning and Melancholia. In *The Standard Edition of the Complete Psychological Works of Sigmund Freud, Volume XIV (1914–1916)*. James Strachey et al., trans. Pp. 237–58. London: The Hogwarth Press.

———. 2003. *Beyond the Pleasure Principle and Other Writings*. John Reddick, trans. London: Penguin.

Friedson, Steven M. 1996. *Dancing Prophets: Musical Experience in Tumbuka Healing*. Chicago: University of Chicago Press.

Geertz, Clifford. 1993[1973]. *The Interpretation of Cultures*. London: Fontana Press.

Gomart, Emilie. 2002. Towards Generous Constraint: Freedom and Coercion in a French Addiction Treatment. *Sociology of Health and Illness* 24(5): 517–49.

Gormsen, Lise Kirstine. 2006. Autonomiens Problematisering: En Refleksion over Autonomibegrebet i en Psykiatrisk Forskningspraksis. *Tidsskrift for Forskning i Sygdom og Samfund* 4(4): 11–31.

Grimshaw, Anna and Amanda Ravetz. 2009. Rethinking Observational Cinema. *Journal of the Royal Anthropological Institute* 15: 538–56.

Hacking, Ian. 1999. *The Social Production of What?* Cambridge, MA: Harvard University Press.

Haraway, Donna J. 1991. Situated Knowledges: The Science Question in Feminism and the Privilege of Partial Perspective. In *Simians, Cyborgs, and Women: The Reinvention of Nature*. Pp. 183–202. New York: Routledge.

Harrington, Anne. 2000a. Introduction. In *The Placebo Effect: An Interdisciplinary Exploration*. Anne Harrington, ed. Pp. 1–11. Cambridge, MA: Harvard University Press.

———. 2000b. Placebo: Conversations at the Disciplinary Borders. In *The Placebo Effect: An Interdisciplinary Exploration*. Anne Harrington, ed. Pp. 208–50. Cambridge, MA: Harvard University Press.

Harrop, Chris. 2002. The Development of Schizophrenia in Late Adolescence. *Current Psychiatry Reports* 4(4): 293–8.

Harrop, Chris and Peter Trower. 2003. *Why Does Schizophrenia Develop at Late Adolescence: A Cognitive-Developmental Approach to Psychosis*. Chichester: Wiley.

Hastrup, Kirsten. 1992. Anthropological Visions: Some Notes on Visual and Textual Authority. In *Film as Ethnography*. Peter I. Crawford and David Turton, eds. Pp. 8–25. Manchester: Manchester University Press.

Healy, David. 1997. *The Antidepressant Era*. Cambridge, MA: Harvard University Press.

———. 2001. Evidence Biased Psychiatry? *Psychiatric Bulletin* 25(8): 290–1.

———. 2002. *The Creation of Psychopharmacology*. Cambridge, MA: Harvard University Press.

———. 2006. The New Medical Oikumene. In *Global Pharmaceuticals: Ethics, Markets, Practices*. Adriana Petryna, Andrew Lakoff, and Arthur Kleinman, eds. Pp. 1–32. Durham, NC: Duke University Press.

Hegel, Georg Wilhelm Friedrich. 2003[1807]. *The Phenomenology of Mind*. New York: Dover Publications.

Helliwell, John, Richard Layard, and Jeffrey Sachs. 2012. *World Happiness Report 2012*. New York: The Earth Insitute, Columbia University.

———. 2016. *World Happiness Report 2016*. New York: Sustainable Development Solutions Network.

———. 2019. *World Happiness Report 2019*. New York: Sustainable Development Solutions Network.

Helweg-Larsen, Karin, Marianne Kastrup, Armando Baez, Esben M. Flachs. 2007. *Etniske Forskelle i Kontaktmønsteret til Psykiatrisk Behandling: Et Registerbaseret Studie*. Copenhagen: Videnscenter for Transkulturel Psykiatri. Retrieved March 28, 2013. www.si-folkesundhed.dk/upload/text-trykklar_samlet.pdf

Henare, Amiria, Martin Holbraad, and Sari Wastell. 2007. Introduction. In *Thinking through Things: Theorising Artefacts Ethnographically*. Amiria Henare, Martin Holbraad, and Sari Wastell, eds. Pp. 1–31. London: Routledge.

Henley, Paul. 2004. Putting Film to Work: Observational Cinema as Practical Ethnography. In *Working Images: Visual Research and Representation in Ethnography*. Sarah Pink, László Kürti, and Ana Isabel Afonso, eds. Pp. 109–30. London: Routledge.

———. 2006. Spirit Possession, Power, and the Absent Presence of Islam: Re-viewing *Les Maîtres Fous*. *Journal of the Royal Anthropological Institute* 12: 731–61.

Hervik, Peter. 2004. The Danish Cultural World of Unbridgeable Differences. *Ethnos* 69(2): 247–67.

———. 2006. The Predictable Responses to the Danish Cartoons. *Global Media and Communication* 2(2): 225–30.

———. 2011. *The Annoying Difference: The Emergence of Danish Neonationalism, Neoracism, and Populism in the Post-1989 World.* New York and Oxford: Berghahn Books.

Herzfeld, Michael. 1992. *The Social Production of Indifference.* Chicago: University of Chicago Press.

Hirschkind, Charles. 2006. *The Ethical Soundscape: Cassette Sermons and Islamic Counterpublics.* New York: Columbia University Press.

———. 2011. Is there a Secular Body? *Cultural Anthropology* 26(4): 633–47.

———. 2012. Experiments in Devotion Online: The Youtube Khuṭba. *International Journal of Middle East Studies* 44: 5–21.

Højer, Lars and Andreas Bandak. 2015. Introduction: The Power of Example. *Journal of the Royal Anthropological Institute* 21(S1): 1–17.

Holbraad, Martin. 2007. The Power of Powder: Multiplicity and Motion in the Divinatory Cosmology of Cuban Ifá (or *Mana*, Again). In *Thinking through Things: Theorising Artefacts Ethnographically.* Amiria Henare, Martin Holbraad and Sari Wastell, eds. Pp. 189–225. London: Routledge.

———. 2012. *Truth in Motion: The Recursive Anthropology of Cuban Divination.* Chicago: Chicago University Press.

Holbraad, Martin and Rane Willerslev. 2007. Transcendental Perspectivism: Anonymous Viewpoints from Inner Asia. *Inner Asia* 9(2): 329–45.

Holenstein, Elmar. 1999. The Zero-Point of Orientation: The Placement of the I in Perceived Space. In *The Body.* Donn Welton, ed. Pp. 57–94. Oxford: Blackwell Publishers.

Hopkins, Nicholas S. 2007. Spirit Mediumship in Upper Egypt. *Anthropos* 102(2): 403–19.

Horner, Robyn. 2005. *Jean-Luc Marion: A Theo-Logical Introduction.* London: Ashgate Publishing Company.

Hubert, Henri and Marcel Mauss. 1964. *Sacrifice: Its Nature and Function.* W. D. Halls, trans. Chicago: The University of Chicago Press.

Huffington Post. 2012. Mother Sara Ege Guilty of Murder of Son Yaseen, 7, Beaten to Death for not Learning Koran. Newspaper article. Retrieved 11 October 2018. www.huffingtonpost.co.uk/2012/12/05/koran-beaten-murder-ege-sara_n_2245077.html

Information. 2005. DFer: Sæt Muslimer i Russiske Fængsler. Newspaper article. Retrieved 11 October 2018. www.information.dk/113012

International Community for Hearing Voices. 2012. What is Intervoice? Retrieved 11 October 2018. www.intervoiceonline.org/about-intervoice

Irving, Andrew. 2013. Into the Gloaming: A Montage of the Senses. In *Transcultural Montage.* Christian Suhr and Rane Willerslev, eds. Pp. 76–95. New York: Berghahn.

———. 2017. *The Art of Life and Death: Radical Aesthetics and Ethnographic Practice.* Chicago: HAU Books.

Jacobsen, Brian Arly. 2007. Muslimer i Danmark: En Kritisk Vurdering af Antalsopgørelser. In *Tørre Tal om Troen: Religionsdemografi i det 21. Århundrede.* Margit Warburg og Brian Jacobsen, eds. Pp. 143–65. Højbjerg: Univers.

———. 2008. Muslimer i Mandtal: Tal, Fordomme og Politik i Europa. *Tidsskrift for Islamforskning* 3(1): 84–110.

Jacobsen, Erling. 1984. *De Psykiske Grundprocesser.* Copenhagen: Centrum.

Jeldoft, Nadia. 2013. The Hypervisibility of Islam. In *Everyday Lived Islam in Europe.* Nathal M. Dessing, Nadia Jeldoft, Jørgen S. Nielsen, and Linda Woodhead, eds. Pp. 28–38. Surrey: Ashgate.

Jensen, Pernille. 2006. *En Helt Anden Hjælp: Recovery i Bruger- og Pårørendeperspektiv.* Copenhagen: Akademisk Forlag.

Johansen, Christoffer and Niels Christian Hvidt, eds. 2003. *Kan Tro Flytte Bjerge?* Copenhagen: Gyldendal.

Johansen, Katrine Schepelern. 2007. Kategorisering i Psykiatrien: Patienter med Anden Etnisk Baggrund end Dansk. In *Intregration: Antropologiske Perspektiver*. Karen Fog Olwig and Karsten Pærregaard, eds. Pp. 155–71. Copenhagen: Museum Tusculanums Forlag.

Johansen, Mette-Louise and Steffen Jensen. 2017. They want us out: Urban Regeneration and the Limits of Integration in the Danish Welfare State. *Critique of Anthropology* 37(3): 297–316.

Jyllandsposten. 2011. Islamisk Gruppe Vækker Afsky. Newspaper article. Retrieved 28 March 2013. http://jyllands-posten.dk/indland/article2578564.ece

Kapferer, Bruce. 2013. Montage and Time: Deleuze, Cinema and a Buddhist Sorcery Rite. In *Transcultural Montage*. Christian Suhr and Rane Willerslev, eds. Pp 20–39. New York: Berghahn.

———. 2014. *2001 and Counting: Kubrick, Nietzsche, and Anthropology*. Chicago: Prickly Paradigm Press.

Karlsson, Bengt. 2009. Pasienterfaringer som Kunnskapsgrunnlag i Psykiatrisk Sykepleie. In *Psykiatrisk Sygepleje*. Niels Buus, ed. Copenhagen: Dansk Sygeplejeråd og Nyt Nordisk Forlag Arnold Busck.

Kassim, Husain. 1971. Existentialist tendencies in Ghazali and Kierkegaard. *Islamic Studies* 10: 103–28.

Kaufmann, Walter. 1965. *Hegel: A Reinterpretation*. New York: Doubleday.

Keane, Webb. 2009. Freedom and Blasphemy: On Indonesian Press Bans and Danish Cartoons. *Public Culture* 21(1): 47–76.

———. 2013. On Spirit Writing: Materialities of Language and the Religious Work of Transduction. *Journal of the Royal Anthropological Institute* 19(1): 1–17.

Kelly, Sean D. 2005. Seeing Things in Merleau-Ponty. In *The Cambridge Companion to Merleau-Ponty*. Taylor Carman and Mark B. N. Hansen, eds. Pp. 74–110. Cambridge: Cambridge University Press.

Kessler, Edward. 2004. *Bound by the Bible: Jews, Christians and the Sacrifice of Isaac*. Cambridge: Cambridge University Press.

Khan, Naveeda. 2006. Of Children and Jinn: An Inquiry into an Unexpected Friendship During Uncertain Times. *Cultural Anthropology* 21(2): 234–64.

Kiener, Wilma. 2008. The Absent and the Cut. *Visual Anthropology* 21: 393–409.

Kierkegaard, Søren. 2005[1843]. *Fear and Trembling*. Alastair Hannay, trans. London: Penguin.

Kiev, Ari. 1962. The Psychotherapeutic Aspects of Primitive Medicine. *Human Organization* 21(1): 25–9.

Kirsch, Irving. 2000. Specifying Non-Specifics: Psychological Mechanisms of Placebo Effects. In *The Placebo Effect: An Interdisciplinary Exploration*. Anne Harrington, ed. Pp. 166–86. Cambridge, MA: Harvard University Press.

———. 2010. *The Emperor's New Drugs: Exploding the Antidepressant Myth*. New York: Basic Books.

Kleinman, Arthur. 1980. *Patients and Healers in the Context of Culture: An Exploration of the Borderland between Anthropology, Medicine, and Psychiatry*. Berkeley: University of California Press.

———. 1988. *The Illness Narratives: Suffering, Healing, and the Human Condition*. New York: Basic Books.

———. 2012. Culture, Bereavement, and Psychiatry. *The Lancet* 379(9816): 608–9.

Klitgaard, Ann-Charlotte. 2009. Recovery: Psykiatrien har brug for nye historier. *Bedre Psykiatri* 2: 7–9.

Köhn, Steffen. 2016. *Mediating Mobility: Visual Anthropology in the Age of Migration*. New York: Wallflower Press.

Kreinath, Jens. 2012. Comment on the Article 'Can Film Show the Invisible: The Work of Montage in Ethnographic Filmmaking'. *Current Anthropology* 53(3): 296–7.

Kühle, Lene. 2006. *Moskeer i Danmark: Islam og Muslimske Bedesteder*. Højbjerg: Forlaget Univers.

Larsen, Birgitte Romme. 2011. Drawing back the Curtains: The Role of Domestic Space in the Social Inclusion and Exclusion of Refugees in Rural Denmark. *Social Analysis* 55(2): 142–58.

Larsen, Timothy. 2014. *The Slain God: Anthropologists and the Christian Faith*. Oxford: Oxford University Press.

Latour, Bruno. 1993. *We Have Never Been Modern*. Catherine Potter, trans. Cambridge, MA: Harvard University Press.

———. 2002. What is Iconoclash? Or is there a World beyond the Image Wars. In *Iconoclash: Beyond the Image Wars in Science, Religion, and Art*. Bruno Latour and Peter Weibel, eds. Pp. 14–37. Cambridge, MA: MIT Press.

———. 2004. Why has Critique Run Out of Steam? From Matters of Fact to Matters of Concern. *Critical Inquiry* 30(2): 225–48.

Lauritsen, Peter. 2011. *Big Brother 2.0: Danmark som Overvågningssamfund*. Copenhagen: Informations Forlag.

Lehmann, Arthur C. and James E. Myers. 1993. The Anthropological Study of Religion: Introduction. In *Magic, Witchcraft, and Religion: An Anthropological Study of the Supernatural*. Arthur C. Lehmann and James E. Myers, eds. Pp. 1–5. Mountain View: Mayfield Publishing Company.

Levinas, Emmanuel. 1979[1961]. *Totality and Infinity: An Essay on Exteriority*. Alphonso Lingis, trans. The Hague: Martinus Nijhoff Publishers.

———. 1985. *Ethics and Infinity: Conversations with Philippe Nemo*. Richard A. Cohen, trans. Pittsburgh: Duquesne University Press.

———. 1987a. *Time and the Other and Additional Essays*. Richard A. Cohen, trans. Pittsburgh: Duquesne University Press.

———. 1987b. *Collected Philosophical Papers*. Alphonso Lingis, trans. Dordrecht: Martinus Nijhoff Publishers.

Levine, Bruce. 2004. Eli Lilly, Zyprexa, and the Bush Family: The Diseasing of our Malaise. *Z Magazine* 17(5). Retrieved 8 March 2013. http://psychrights.org/articles/LevineLillyandBush.htm

Lévi-Strauss, Claude. 1983[1964]. *The Raw and the Cooked: Mythologiques. Vol. 1*. John and Doreen Weightman, trans. Chicago: University of Chicago Press.

———. 1993[1963]. The Sorcerer and His Magic. In *Magic, Witchcraft, and Religion: An Anthropological Study of the Supernatural*. Arthur C. Lehmann and James E. Myers, eds. Pp. 169–78. Mountain View: Mayfield Publishing Company.

———. 2001[1978]. *Myth and Meaning*, London: Routledge.

Lindekilde, Lasse. 2010. Forebyggelse af Radikalisering, Miskendelse og Muslimsk Minoritetsidentitet. *Tidsskrift for Islamforskning* 2010(2): 7–29.

Lovat, Terry and Inna Semetsky. 2009. Practical Mysticism and Deleuze's Ontology of the Virtual. *Cosmos and History: The Journal of Natural and Social Philosophy* 5(2): 236–49.

Luhrmann, Tanya. 2000. *Of Two Minds: The Growing Disorder in American Psychiatry*. New York: Vintage Books.

———. 2012a. Living with Voices: A New Way to Deal with Disturbing Voices Offers Hope for Those with Other Forms of Psychosis. *The American Scholar* 81(3): 48. Retrieved 20 November 2016. https://theamericanscholar.org/living-with-voices/#.WhLu-rbMzMU

———. 2012b. *When God Talks Back: Understanding the American Evangelical Relationship with God*. New York: Alfred Knopf.

———. 2016. Understanding the Work of Faith. In *Faith in Anthropology: A Symposium on Timothy Larsen's The Slain God*. Brian Howell, et al. *The Cambridge Journal of Anthropology* 34(2): 147–9.

Maarouf. Mohammed. 2007. *Jinn Eviction as a Discourse of Power: A Multidisciplinary Approach to Moroccan Magical Beliefs and Practices*. Leiden: Brill Academic Publishers.

MacDougall, David. 1998. *Transcultural Cinema*. Princeton: Princeton University Press.

———. 2006. *The Corporeal Image: Film, Ethnography, and the Senses*. Princeton: Princeton University Press.

Mahmood, Saba. 2005. *Politics of Piety: The Islamic Revival and the Feminist Subject*. Princeton: Princeton University Press.

———. 2009. Religious Reason and Secular Affect: An Incommensurable Divide? *Critical Inquiry* 35(4): 836–62.

Malinowski, Bronislaw. 2004[1948]. *Magic, Science and Religion and Other Essays.* With introduction by Robert Redfield. Whitefish, MT: Kessinger Publishing.

Marcus, George E. 1994. The Modernist Sensibility in Recent Ethnographic Writing and the Cinematic Metaphor of Montage. In *Visualizing Theory: Selected Essays from V.A.R. 1990–1994.* Lucien Taylor, ed. Pp. 37–53. New York: Routledge.

———. 1998. The Uses of Complicity in the Changing Mise-en-Scène of Anthropological Fieldwork. In *Ethnography through Thick and Thin.* Pp. 105–32. Princeton: Princeton University Press.

———. 2013. Afterword: The Traffic in Montage, Then and Now. In *Transcultural Montage.* Christian Suhr and Rane Willerslev, eds. Pp. 302–7. New York: Berghahn.

Marion, Jean-Luc. 2002. *In Excess: Studies of Saturated Phenomena.* Robyn Horner and Vincent Berraud, trans. New York: Fordham University Press.

Marks, Laura U. 2000. *The Skin of the Film: Intercultural Cinema, Embodiment, and the Senses.* London: Duke University Press.

———. 2010. *Enfoldment and Infinity: An Islamic Genealogy of New Media Art.* Cambridge, MA: Massachusetts Institute of Technology.

Marx, Karl. 1975[1844]. Introduction: A Contribution to the Critique of Hegel's Philosophy of the Right. In *Early Writings.* Pp. 244–57. Harmondsworth: Penguin Books.

Marx, Karl and Frederich Engels. 1988[1844]. *Economic and Philosophical Manuscripts of 1844 and the Communist Manifesto.* Martin Milligan, trans. New York: Prometheus Books.

Mattingly, Cheryl. 1998. *Healing Dramas and Clinical Plots: The Narrative Structure of Experience.* Cambridge: Cambridge University Press.

———. 2010. Moral Willing as Narrative Re-Envisioning. In *Toward an Anthropology of the Will.* Keith Murphy and Jason Throop, eds. Pp. 50–69. Stanford: Stanford University Press.

———. 2012. Two Virtue Ethics and the Anthropology of Morality. *Anthropological Theory* 12(2): 161–84.

McGlashan, T., R. Zipusky, D. Perkins, J. Addington, T. Miller, S. Woods, K. Hawkins, R. Hoffman, A. Preda, I. Epstein, D. Addington, S. Lindborg, Q. Trzaskoma, M. Tohen, and A. Breier. 2006. Randomized, Double-Blind Trial of Olanzapine Versus Placebo in Patients Prodromally Symptomatic for Psychosis. *American Journal of Psychiatry* 163(5): 790–9.

Mead, Margaret and Gregory Bateson. 1977. On the Use of the Camera in Anthropology. *Studies in the Anthropology of Visual Communication* 4(2): 78–80.

Merleau-Ponty, Maurice. 1964[1948]. *Sense and Nonsense.* Hubert L. Dreyfus and Patricia Allen Dreyfus, trans. Evanston, IL: Northwestern University Press.

———. 1976. Philosophy and Non-Philosophy since Hegel. *Telos* 29: 43–105.

———. 1988. *In Praise of Philosophy and Other Essays.* Evanston, IL: Northwestern University Press.

———. 1997[1964]. *The Visible and the Invisible: Followed by Working Notes.* Alphonso Lingis, trans. Evanston: Northwestern University Press.

———. 2000. Eye and Mind. In *The Primacy of Perception: And Other Essays on Phenomenological Psychology, the Philosophy of Art, History and Politics.* James M. Edie, ed. William Cobb, trans. Pp. 159–90. Evanston: Northwestern University Press.

———. 2002[1945]. *Phenomenology of Perception.* Colin Smith, trans. New York: Routledge.

Metcalf, Peter. 2002. *They Lie, We Lie: Getting on with Anthropology.* London: Routledge.

Ministries of the Interior, Health, and Social Affairs. 2005. Respekt, Faglighed, Ansvar: Fælles Værdier i Indsatsen for Mennesker med en Sindslidelse. Policy paper. Retrieved 14 April 2019. www.sum.dk/Aktuelt/Publikationer/Faelles-vaedier-i-indsatsen-for-mennekser-med-en-sindslidelse-dec-2005.aspx

Ministry of Social Affairs. 2011. *Liste over ghettoområder pr. 1. januar 2011.* Policy Paper. Retrieved 28 March 2013. www.sm.dk/data/Dokumentertilnyheder/2011/ghettoomr%C3%A5der_pr_1_januar.pdf

Ministry of Transport, Building, and Housing. 2016. *Liste over ghettoområder pr. 1. december 2016*. Policy paper. Retrieved 7 November 2017. www.trm.dk/da/publikationer/2016/liste-over-ghettoomraader

Mittermaier, Amira. 2011. *Dreams that Matter: Egyptian Landscapes of the Imagination*. Berkeley: University of California Press.

Nathan, Tobie and Isabelle Stengers. 2018. *Doctors and Healers*. Cambridge, UK: Polity Press.

Nielsen, Maria Rebecca, Anne Marie Mikkelsen, and Jørgen Aagaard. 2009. *Styr på Stemmerne: Gruppetilbud til Stemmehørere*. Aarhus: Center for Psykiatrisk Forskning, Janssen-Cilag.

Norredam, Marie, A. Garcia Lopez, N. Keiding, and A. Krasnik. 2009. Risk of Mental Disorders in Refugees and Native Danes: A Register-Based Retrospective Cohort Study. *Social Psychiatry and Psychiatric Epidemiology* 44: 1023–9.

OED. 2019. *Oxford English Dictionary Online*. Oxford: Oxford University Press. Retrieved 15 January 2019. www.oed.com

Ohnuma, Reiko. 2007. *Head, Eyes, Flesh, and Blood: Giving Away the Body in Indian Buddhist Literature*. New York: Columbia University Press.

OPUS. 2007. Opsøgende Behandling af Psykotiske Unge. Retrieved 11 October 2018. https://viden.sl.dk/media/5888/opus-danske-regioern.pdf

Ortner, Sherry B. 1984. Theory in Anthropology since the Sixties. *Comparative Studies in Society and History* 26(1): 126–66.

———. 2006. *Anthropology and Social Theory: Culture, Power, and the Acting Subject*. Durham, NC: Duke University Press.

Otto, Ton. 1997. Informed Participation and Participating Informants. *Canberra Anthropology* 20(1–2): 96–108.

Otto, Ton and Poul Pedersen. 2005. Disentangling Traditions: Culture, Agency and Power. In *Tradition and Agency. Tracing Cultural Continuity and Invention*. Ton Otto and Poul Pedersen, eds. Pp. 11–49. Aarhus: Aarhus University Press.

Pandolfo, Stefania. 1997. *Impasse of the Angels: Scenes from a Moroccan Space of Memory*. Chicago: University of Chicago Press.

———. 2007. The Burning: Finitude and the Politico-Theological Imagination of Illegal Migration. *Anthropological Theory* 7(3): 329–63.

———. 2011. Clad in Mourning: Violence, Subjugation and the Struggle of the Soul. In *Review of Women Studies*. Pp. 25–39. Excerpt from keynote address held at the IWS Conference, Birzeit University, March 2010.

———. 2018. *Knot of the Soul: Madness, Psychiatry, Islam*. Chicago: University of Chicago Press.

Parker, Gordon, Ian M. Anderson, and Peter Haddad. 2003. Clinical Trials of Antidepressant Medications are Producing Meaningless Results. *The British Journal of Psychiatry* 183(2): 102–4.

Pattison, E. Mansell. 1977. Psychosocial Interpretations of Exorcism. *Journal of Operational Psychiatry* 8(2): 5–21.

Pedersen, Morten Axel. 2011. *Not Quite Shamans: Spirit Worlds and Political Lives in Northern Mongolia*. Ithaca, NY: Cornell University Press.

Pelkmans, Mathijs, ed. 2013. *Ethnographies of Doubt: Faith and Uncertainty in Contemporary Societies*. New York: I. B. Tauris.

Petersen, Lone, Merete Nordentoft, Pia Jeppesen, Johan Øhlenschlæger, Anne Thorup, Torben Østergaard Christensen, Gertrud Krarup, Jytte Dahlstrøm, Bodil Haastrup, and Per Jørgensen. 2005. Improving 1-Year Outcome in First-Episode Psychosis: OPUS Trial. *The British Journal of Psychiatry* 187: 98–103.

Petryna, Adriana and Arthur Kleinman. 2006. The Pharmaceutical Nexus. In *Global Pharmaceuticals: Ethics, Markets, Practices*. Adriana Petryna, Andrew Lakoff, and Arthur Kleinman, eds. Pp. 1–32. Durham, NC: Duke University Press.

Philips, Bilal. 2007. *The Exorcist Tradition in Islam*. Birmingham: Al-Hidaayah Publishing.

Politiken. 2012. Marie Krarup: Vi er i krig med den islamiske civilization [Marie Krarup: We are at War with the Islamic Civilisation]. Newspaper article. Retrieved 15 January

2019. https://politiken.dk/indland/politik/art5423431/Marie-Krarup-Vi-er-i-krig-med-den-islamiske-civilisation

———. 2013. Jobopslag: Folkekirke søger præst som tror på Gud [Church Seeks Priest who Believes in God]. Newspaper article. Retrieved 28 March 2013. http://politiken.dk/indland/ECE1874334/jobopslag-folkekirke-soeger-praest—som-tror-paa-gud/

Quist, Pia. 2000. Ny Københavnsk 'Multietnolekt'. *Danske Talesprog* 1: 143–211.

Rabinow, Paul. 1996. *Making PCR: A Story of Biotechnology*. Chicago: University of Chicago Press.

Rasmussen, Klavs Serup. 2006. Psykiatribrugere må acceptere at få sukkersyge. *Outsideren* 58: 18–19. Retrieved 8 March 2013. www.outsideren.dk/wp-content/uploads/2009/12/2006_nummer58.pdf#page=18

Ray, Wayne A., Cecilia P. Chung, Katherine T. Murray, Kathi Hall, and C. Michael Stein. 2009. Atypical Antipsychotic Drugs and the Risk of Sudden Cardiac Death. *New England Journal of Medicine* 360(3): 225–35.

Region Midtjylland. 2009. Politik for Samarbejde mellem Psykisk Syge, Pårørende og Personale i Behandlings-og Socialpsykiatrien. Policy paper. Retrieved 4 March 2013. www.regionmidtjylland.dk/politik/regionsrådets+møder/visdagsorden?file=29–04–2009/Aaben_dagsorden/Bilag/Punkt_6_Bilag_2______.PDF

Ringgaard, Anne. 2012. Ingen gider forske i indvandreres sundhed. Interview with Allan Krasnik. *Videnskab.dk*. Retrieved 28 March 2013. http://videnskab.dk/krop-sundhed/ingen-gider-forske-i-indvandreres-sundhed

Robbins, Joel. 2015. Ritual, Value, and Example: On the Perfection of Cultural Representations. *Journal of the Royal Anthropological Institute* 21(S1): 18–29.

Roberts, Graham. 2000. *The Man with the Movie Camera*. London: I. B. Tauris.

Romme, Marius and Sandra Escher. 2000. *Making Sense of Voices: A Guide for Mental Health Professionals Working with Voice-Hearers*. London: Mind Publications.

Rorty, Richard. 1991a. *Consequences of Pragmatism*. New York: Harvester Wheatsheaf.

———. 1991b. *Objectivity, Relativism and Truth*. Cambridge: Cambridge University Press.

Rose, Nikolas. 2003. Neurochemical Selves. *Society* 41(1): 46–59.

———. 2018. *Our Psychiatric Future: The Politics of Mental Health*. Cambridge: Polity.

Rothenberg, Celia. 2004. *Spirits of Palestine: Gender, Society and Stories of the Jinn*. Maryland: Lexington Press.

Rothman, William. 1997. *Documentary Film Classics*. Cambridge: Cambridge University Press.

Rouch, Jean. 2003. The Camera and Man. In *Principles of Visual Anthropology*. Paul Hockings, ed. Pp. 79–98. New York: Mouton de Gruyter.

Russell, Catherine. 1999. *Experimental Ethnography: The Work of Film in the Age of Video*. Durham, NC, and London: Duke University Press.

Rytter, Mikkel. 2010a. The Family of Denmark and the Aliens: Kinship Images in Danish Integration Politics. *Ethnos* 75(3): 301–22.

———. 2010b. In-laws and Outlaws: Black Magic among Pakistani Migrants in Denmark. *Journal of the Royal Anthropological Institute* 16(1): 46–63.

———. 2018. Writing against Integration: Danish Imaginaries of Culture, Race and Belonging. *Ethnos*, DOI: 10.1080/00141844.2018.1458745.

Rytter, Mikkel and Marianne Pedersen. 2014. A Decade of Suspicion: Islam and Muslims in Denmark after 9/11. *Ethnic and Racial Studies* 37(13): 2303–21.

Said, Edward W. 1995. *Orientalism: Western Conceptions of the Orient*. London: Penguin.

Safer, Daniel J. 2002. Design and Reporting Modifications in Industry-Sponsored Comparative Psychopharmacology Trials. *The Journal of Nervous and Mental Disease* 190(9): 583–92.

Samvirket i Gellerup og Toveshøj. 2016. *Fakta og Tal*. Retrieved 17 September 2017. http://samvirket.dk/fakta

Sartre, Jean Paul 2000[1943]. *Being and Nothingness: An Essay on Phenomenological Ontology*. Hazel E. Barnes, trans. Oxon: Routledge.

Schäuble, Michaela. 2016a. Mining Imagination: Ethnographic Approaches Beyond the Written Word. *Anthrovision* 4(2): 1–11.

———. 2016b. Images of Ecstasy and Affliction: The Camera as Instrument for Researching and Reproducing Choreographies of Deviance in a Southern Italian Spider Possession Cult. *Anthrovision* 4(2): 1–28.

Schielke, Samuli. 2010. Second Thoughts about the Anthropology of Islam, or How to Make Sense of Grand Schemes in Everyday Life. Berlin: Zentrum Moderner Orient Working Papers.

———. 2019. *The Power of God: Four Proposals for an Anthropological Engagement*. ZMO Programmatic Texts 13, Pp. 1–20. Berlin: Leibniz-Zentrum Moderner Orient (ZMO).

Schilbrack, Kevin. 2005. Religion, Models of, and Reality: Are we Through with Geertz? *Journal of the American Academy of Religion* 73: 429–52.

Schmidt, Anders Legarth. 2013. Endnu En Patient Dør På Lukket Psykiatrisk Afdeling. Newspaper article. *Politiken*. Retrieved 11 October 2018. http://politiken.dk/indland/ECE1914909/endnu-en-patient-doer-paa-lukket-psykiatrisk-afdeling/

Schmidt, Garbi, Birgitte Schepelern Johansen, and Dorthe Høvids Possing. 2008. Foreword. In *Research on Islam Repositioned: New Agendas in the Study of Islam and Muslims in a Politicised Research Field*. Special issue of *Tidsskrift for Islamforskning* 2: 3–4.

Schwartz, Louis-Georges. 2005. Typewriter: Free Indirect Discourse in Deleuze's Cinema. *SubStance* 34(3): 107–35.

Scott, James C. 1990. *Domination and the Arts of Resistance: Hidden Transcripts*. New Haven: Yale University Press.

———. 1998. *Seeing like a State: How Certain Schemes to Improve the Human Condition have Failed*. New Haven: Yale University Press.

Sedgwick, Mark. 2006. *Islam and Muslims: A Guide to Diverse Experience in a Modern World*. Boston: Intercultural Press.

———. 2010. Contextualizing Salafism. *Tidskrift for Islamforskning* 1: 75–81.

———. 2014. Introduction: Families, Governments, Schools, Alternatice Spaces and the Making of European Muslims. In *Making European Muslims: Religious Socialization and the Formation of Identities among Muslim Children and Young Muslims in Western Europe*. Mark Sedgwick, ed. Pp. 1–20. London: Routledge.

———. 2016. *Western Sufism: From the Abbasids to the New Age*. Oxford: Oxford University Press.

Severi, Carlo. 2002. Memory, Reflexivity and Belief: Reflections on the Ritual Use of Language. *Social Anthropology* 10(1): 23–40.

Shariati, Ali. 1979. *On the Sociology of Islam: Lectures by Ali Shariati*. Hamid Algar, trans. New York: Mizan Press.

Simonsen, Erik. 2012. Den Etiske Fordring i Psykiatrien. Newspaper article. *Politiken*. Retrieved 11 October 2018. http://politiken.dk/debat/kroniken/ECE1807137/den-etiske-fordring-i-psykiatrien/

Sjørslev, Inger. 2002. Forestillinger om Folket. In *Folkets Repræsentanter: Et Antropologisk Blik på Folketinget*. Finn Sivert Nielsen and Inger Sjørslev, eds. Pp. 9–34. Aarhus: Aarhus Universitetsforlag.

Skovgaard-Petersen, Jakob. 2016. Der er forskel på had-, svovl- og reformprædikanter. Online opinion article. *Danmarks Radio*. Retrieved 11 October 2018. www.dr.dk/nyheder/kultur/tro/islamforsker-der-er-forskel-paa-had-svovl-og-reformpraedikanter

Slater, Tom. 2010. Ghetto Blasting: On Loïc Wacquant's Urban Outcasts. *Urban Geography* 31(2): 162–8.

Sobchack, Vivian. 1992. *The Address of the Eye: A Phenomenology of Film Experience*. Princeton: Princeton University Press.

Spiro, Melford E. 1966. Religion: Problems of Definition and Explanation. In *Anthropological Approaches to the Study of Religion*. Michael Banton, ed. Pp. 85–126. London: Tavistock Publications.

Stage, Carsten. 2011. *Tegningekrisen: Som Mediebegivenhed og Danskhedskamp*. Aarhus: Aarhus Universitetsforlag.

Steinbock, Anthony J. 2007. *Phenomenology and Mysticism: The Verticality of Religious Experience*. Bloomington, IN: Indiana University Press.

Stoller, Paul. 1984. Eye, Mind and Word in Anthropology. *L'Homme* 24: 91–114.

Suhr, Christian. 2014. Brainwashed at School: Deprogramming the Secular among Young Neo-Orthodox Muslims in Denmark. In *Making European Muslims: Religious Socialization Among Young Muslims in Scandinavia and Western Europe*. Mark Sedgwick, ed. Pp. 249–68. London: Routledge.

———. 2015. The Failed Image and the Possessed: Examples of Invisibility in Visual Anthropology and Islam. *Journal of the Royal Anthropological Society* 21(1): 96–112.

———. 2016. Livet i moskeerne er langt mere, end hvad vi ser i TV [Life in the Mosques is More Than we See on TV]. Opinion article. *Politiken*. Retrieved 11 October 2018. https://politiken.dk/debat/kroniken/art5614897/Livet-i-moskeerne-er-langt-mere-end-hvad-vi-ser-i-tv

———. 2017. Islamic Exorcism and the Cinema Fist: Analyzing Exorcism among Danish Muslims through the Prism of Film. *Contemporary Islam*. https://doi.org/10.1007/s11562–017–0394–6

———. 2018. Camera Monologue: Cultural Critique beyond Collaboration, Participation and Dialogue. *Journal of Visual Anthropology* 31: 376–93.

Suhr, Christian and Kirstine Sinclair. 2016. Fakta og Fiktion om muslimer i danske medier [Facts and Fictions about Danish Muslims in Danish Media]. *Tidsskrift for Islamforskning* 10(1): 134–48.

Suhr, Christian and Rane Willerslev. 2012. Can Film Show the Invisible: The Work of Montage in Ethnographic Filmmaking. *Current Anthropology* 53(3): 282–301.

———. 2013. *Transcultural Montage*. New York: Berghahn.

Suhr, Christian, Hjarn von Zernichow Borberg, Kirstine Sinclair, and Niels Valdemar Vinding. 2017. Cavling-nomineret tv-dokumentar er unuanceret og menings forvridende [Cavling-nominated TV Documentary is One-sided and Misleading]. Opinion article. *Politiken*. Retrieved 11 October 2018. https://politiken.dk/debat/kroniken/art5771535/Cavling-nomineret-dokumentar-er-unuanceret-og-meningsforvridende

Tambiah, Stanley Jeyaraya. 1990. *Magic, Science, Religion, and the Scope of Rationality*. Cambridge: Cambridge University Press.

Tamen, Miguel. 2001. *Friends of Interpretable Objects*. Massachusetts, MA: Harvard University Press.

Taneja, Anand Vivek. 2017. *Jinnealogy: Time, Islam, and Ecological Thought in the Medieval Ruins of Delhi*. Stanford, CA: Stanford University Press.

Taussig, Michael. 1980. *The Devil and Commodity Fetishism in South America*. Chapel Hill: University of North Carolina Press.

———. 1986. *Shamanism, Colonialism, and the Wild Man: A Study in Terror and Healing*. Chicago: University of Chicago Press.

———. 1993. *Mimesis and Alterity: A Particular History of the Senses*. London: Routledge.

———. 1999. *Defacement: Public Secrecy and the Labor of the Negative*. Stanford: Stanford University Press.

Taylor, Charles. 1990. *Philosophy and the Human Sciences: Philosophical Papers 2*. Cambridge: Cambridge University Press.

Taymiyah, S. I. I. 2007[1263–1328 C.E.]. *Essay on the Jinn*. Bilal Philips, ed. and trans. Riyadh: International Islamic Publishing House.

Thorup, A., L. Petersen, P. Jeppesen, J. Øhlenschlæger, T. Christensen, G. Krarup, P. Jørgensen, and M. Nordentoft. 2005. Integrated Treatment Ameliorates Negative Symptoms in First Episode Psychosis: Results from the Danish Opus Trial. *Schizophrenia Research* 79: 95–105.

Tiihonen, Jari, Jouko Lönnqvist, Kristian Wahlbeck, Timo Klaukka, Antti Tanskanen, and Jari Haukka. 2006. Antidepressants and the Risk of Suicide, Attempted Suicide, and Overall Mortality in a Nationwide Cohort. *Archives of General Psychiatry* 63(12): 1358–67.

Tomlinson, Matt. 2014. Bringing Kierkegaard into Anthropology: Repetition, Absurdity, and Curses in Fiji. *American Ethnologist* 41: 163–75.

Transparency International. 2016. *Corruption Perceptions Index 2016*. Berlin: Transparency International.

Trinh, T. Minh-Ha. 1991. *When the Moon Waxes Red: Representation, Gender and Cultural Politics*. New York: Routledge.

Turner, Edith. 1989. From Shamans to Healers: The Survival of an Inupiaq Eskimo Skill. *Anthropologica* 31(1): 3–24.

———. 1992. *Experiencing Ritual: A New Interpretation of African Healing*. Philadelphia: University of Pennsylvania Press.

———. 1993. The Reality of Spirits: A Tabooed or Permitted Field of Study. *Anthropology of Consciousness* 4(1): 9–12.

———. 2006. Advances in the Study of Spirit Experience: Drawing Together Many Threads. *Anthropology of Consciousness* 17(2): 33–61.

Turner, Erick H., Daniel Knoepflmacher, and Lee Shapley. 2012. Publication Bias in Antipsychotic Trials: An Analysis of Efficacy comparing the Published Literature to the US Food and Drug Administration Database. *PLOS Medicine* 9(3): 1–17.

Turner, Victor. 1967. *The Forest of Symbols: Aspects of Ndembu Ritual*. Ithaca: Cornell University Press.

US Department of Justice. 2009. Eli Lilly and Company Agrees to Pay $1.415 Billon to Resolve Allegations of Off-label Promotion of Zyprexa. Retrieved 8 March 2013. www.justice.gov/opa/pr/2009/January/09-civ-038.html

Vacher, Mark. 2010. Looking at Houses, Searching for Homes: An Anthropological Analysis of the Relationship between Danish Homeowners and their Houses. *Ethnologia Scandinavica* 40: 52–67.

van Beek, Martijn. 2012. Enlightened Democracy: Normative Secularism and Spiritual Authority on the Margins of Indian Politics. In *Varieties of Secularism in Asia: Anthropological Explorations of Religion, Politics and the Spiritual*. Nils Bubandt and Martijn van Beek, eds. Pp. 75–100. London: Routledge.

van der Geest, Sjaak. 2005. 'Sacraments' in the Hospital: Exploring the Magic and Religion of Recovery. *Anthropology and Medicine* 12(2): 135–50.

Vaughan, Dai. 1992. The Aesthetics of Ambiguity. In *Film as Ethnography*. Peter I. Crawford and David Turton, eds. Pp. 99–115. Manchester: Manchester University Press.

Vertov, Dziga. 1984. Kinoks: A Revolution. In *Kino-Eye: The Writings of Dziga Vertov*. Annette Michelson, ed. Pp. 11–20. Berkeley: University of California Press.

Videnscenter for Transkulturel Psykiatri. 2012. *Transkulturelle Patienter*. Retrieved 28 March 2013. www.vftp.dk/temaer/fakta%20og%20tal/transkulturelle_patienter.html

Vigh, Henrik and Simon Turner. 2007. Indledning: Usynlighed. *Den Ny Verden Tidsskrift for International Studier* 40(2): 7–14.

Vinding, Niels Valdemar. 2016. The Question of Sharīʿa in Denmark. Blog. Cambridge: Harvard Law School. Retrieved 7 November 2017. https://shariasource.blog/2016/08/03/264/

Viveiros de Castro, Eduardo. 2011. Zeno and the Art of Anthropology: Of Lies, Beliefs, Paradoxes, and Other Truths. *Common Knowledge* 17(1): 128–45.

Wacquant, Loïc. 2008. Ghettos and Anti-Ghettos: An Anatomy of the New Urban Poverty. *Thesis Eleven* 94(1): 113–18.

Wahhab, S. I. M. Abdul. 1996[1703–1792 C.E.]. *The Book of Monotheism*. Riyadh: Darussalam.

Waltorp, Karen. 2018. Intimacy, Concealment and Unconscious Optics: Filmmaking with Young Muslim Women in Copenhagen. *Journal of Visual Anthropology* 31: 394–407.

Weiner, James. 1997. Televisualist Anthropology: Representation, Aesthetics, Politics. *Current Anthropology* 38: 197–235.

White, Adrian. 2006. *University of Leicester Produces the First-ever World Map of Happiness*. Press release. Leicester: University of Leicester. Retrieved 28 March 2013. www2.le.ac.uk/ebulletin/news/press-releases/2000–2009/2006/07/nparticle.2006–07–28.2448323827

Whyte, Susan Reynolds. 1997. *Questioning Misfortune: The Pragmatics of Uncertainty in Eastern Uganda*. Cambridge: Cambridge University Press.

Wikan, Unni. 1991. *Behind the Veil in Arabia: Women in Oman*. Chicago: University of Chicago Press.

Willerslev, Rane. 2007. *Soul Hunters: Hunting, Animism and Personhood among the Siberian Yukaghirs*. Berkeley: University of California Press.

———. 2009a. To have the World at a Distance: Reconsidering the Significance of Vision for Social Anthropology. In *Skilled Visions: Between Apprenticeship and Standards*. Cristina Grassini, ed. Pp. 23–46. London: Berghahn.

———. 2009b. The Optimal Sacrifice: A Study of Voluntary Death among the Siberian Chukchi. *American Ethnologist* 36(4): 693–704.

———. 2013a. Taking Animism Seriously, but Perhaps not too Seriously? *Religion and Society* 4(1): 41–57.

———. 2013b. God on Trial: Human Sacrifice, Trickery and Faith. *HAU: Journal of Ethnographic Theory* 3(1): 140–54.

Willerslev, Rane and Christian Suhr. 2018. Is There a Place for Faith in Anthropology? Religion, Reason, and the Ethnographer's Divine Revelation. *HAU: Journal of Ethnographic Theory* 8(1–2): 65–78.

Willerslev, Rane and Morten Axel Pedersen. 2010. Joking the Cosmos into the Right Shape in North Asia. In *Experiments in Holism: Theory and Practice in Contemporary Anthropology*. Ton Otto and Nils Bubandt, eds. Pp. 262–78. West Sussex: Wiley-Blackwell.

Wyschogrod, Edith. 2002. Language and Alterity in the Thought of Levinas. In *The Cambridge Companion to Levinas*. Simon Critchley and Robert Bernasconi, eds. Pp. 188–205. Cambridge: Cambridge University Press.

Young, Allan. 2011. Self, Brain, Microbe, and the Vanishing Commissar. *Science, Technology, and Human Values* 36(5): 638–61.

Zola, Irving Kenneth. 1973. Pathways to the Doctor: From Person to Patient. *Social Science and Medicine* 7(9): 677–89.

Zuckerman, Phil. 2008. *Society without God: What the Least Religious Nations Can Tell us about Contentment*. New York: New York University Press.

## Films and media

Aaltonen, Jouko. 2001. *Kusum*. 69 min. Helsinki: ILLUME.

Al-Awlaki, Anwar. 2010. *The Hereafter*. Collection of 22 lectures. Retrieved 4 March 2013. www.kalamullah.com/anwar-alawlaki.html

Bateson, Gregory and Margaret Mead. 1952. *Childhood Rivalry in Bali and New Guinea*. 17 min. New York: Penn State Media.

Connor, Linda, Patsy Asch, and Timothy Asch. 1980. *Jero on Jero: A Balinese Trance Seance Observed*. 48 min. Watertown: DER.

Deren, Maya. 1985. *Divine Horsemen: The Living Gods of Haiti*. 52 min. New York: Mystic Fire Video.

Eisenstein, Sergei M. 1928. *October: Ten Days that Shook the World*. 104 min. Moscow: Sovkino.

Herzog, Werner. 1993. *Bells from the Deep: Faith and Superstition in Russia*. 60 min. Vienna: Werner Herzog Filmproduktion.

Khan, Nouman Ali. 2009. *Literary Characteristics of the Quran*. YouTube lecture. 118 min. Retrieved 7 March 2013. www.youtube.com/watch?v=aWUy_luMqoQ

Kildea, Gary and Andrea Simon. 2005. *Koriams Law and the Dead who Govern*. 110 min. Canberra: ANU RSPAS Film Unit.

Rouch, Jean. 1955. *Les Maîtres Fous*. 24 min. Paris: Films de la Pléiade.

———. 1967. *Jaguar*. 93 min. Paris: Les Films de la Pléiade.

Rouch, Jean and Edgar Morin. 1961. *Chronicle of a Summer*. 85 min. Paris: Argos Films.

Suhr, Christian and Mette Bahnsen. 2005. *Want a Camel, Yes?* 36 min. Aarhus: Persona Film.

Thyrri, Irene and Martin Kjær Jensen. 2016. *Moskeerne bag sløret* [The Mosques behind the Veil]. TV documentary, 4 episodes. Aarhus: Filmkompagniet and TV2.

Trinh, T. Minh-ha. 1982. *Reassemblage*. 40 min. New York: Women Make Movies.

Vachani, Nilita. 1990. *Eyes of Stone*. 91 min. New Delhi: FilmSixteen and Doordarshan.

Vertov, Dziga. 1929. *Man with a Movie Camera*. 68 min. Kiev: VUFKU.

# Index